Report of Investigations 9673

Strengthening Existing 20-psi Mine Ventilation Seals With Carbon Fiber-Reinforced Polymer Reinforcement

By Eric S. Weiss and Samuel P. Harteis, P.E.

DEPARTMENT OF HEALTH AND HUMAN SERVICES
Centers for Disease Control and Prevention
National Institute for Occupational Safety and Health
Pittsburgh Research Laboratory
Pittsburgh, PA

January 2008

Disclaimer

Mention of any company or product does not constitute endorsement by the National Institute for Occupational Safety and Health (NIOSH). In addition, citations to Web sites external to NIOSH do not constitute NIOSH endorsement of the sponsoring organizations or their programs or products. Furthermore, NIOSH is not responsible for the content of these Web sites.

Ordering Information

To receive documents or other information about occupational safety and health topics, contact NIOSH at

> Telephone: **1–800–CDC–INFO** (1–800–232–4636)
> TTY: 1–888–232–6348
> e-mail: cdcinfo@cdc.gov

> or visit the NIOSH Web site at **www.cdc.gov/niosh**.

For a monthly update on news at NIOSH, subscribe to NIOSH *eNews* by visiting **www.cdc.gov/niosh/eNews**.

DHHS (NIOSH) Publication No. 2008–106

January 2008

SAFER • HEALTHIER • PEOPLE™

CONTENTS

ILLUSTRATIONS

CONTENTS—Continued

TABLES

ACRONYMS AND ABBREVIATIONS USED IN THIS REPORT

ASTM	American Society for Testing and Materials
CFR	Code of Federal Regulations
CFRP	carbon fiber-reinforced polymer
DG	data-gathering
LVDT	linear variable displacement transducer
MSHA	Mine Safety and Health Administration
NIOSH	National Institute for Occupational Safety and Health
NMA	National Mining Association
LLEM	Lake Lynn Experimental Mine
PRL	Pittsburgh Research Laboratory (NIOSH)

UNIT OF MEASURE ABBREVIATIONS USED IN THIS REPORT

cfm	cubic foot per minute
ft	foot
ft^2	square foot
ft^3	cubic foot
gal	gallon
hr	hour
Hz	hertz
in	inch
in H_2O	inch of water
J	joule
lb	pound
lb/ft^3	pound per cubic foot
m	meter
min	minute
ms	millisecond
psi	pound-force per square inch
sec	second
°C	degree Celsius
°F	degree Fahrenheit

STRENGTHENING EXISTING 20-psi MINE VENTILATION SEALS WITH CARBON FIBER-REINFORCED POLYMER REINFORCEMENT

By Eric S. Weiss[1] and Samuel P. Harteis, P.E.[2]

ABSTRACT

The National Mining Association and the Mine Safety and Health Administration requested that the National Institute for Occupational Safety and Health (NIOSH) conduct full-scale evaluations of a recently developed carbon fiber-reinforced polymer (CFRP) reinforcement technique for upgrading existing mine ventilation seals to withstand an explosion pressure of 50 psi or greater. The evaluation was conducted in the NIOSH Pittsburgh Research Laboratory's Lake Lynn Experimental Mine (LLEM) near Fairchance, PA. The purpose of the evaluation was to determine the blast resistance of the CFRP reinforcement technique, designed to increase the strength of two types of existing 20-psi-rated in situ mine ventilation seals.

Two candidate ventilation seals were selected to represent the 20-psi alternative seal designs typical of those used in mines prior to July 2006. Installed within the LLEM were (1) a 4-ft-thick pumpable cementitious foam seal using material with a designed 150- to 200-psi average compressive strength at 28 days and (2) a 24-in-thick, low-density cementitious block seal with a center pilaster and keyed to the floor and ribs. The materials necessary for the CFRP reinforcement technique were then installed on the outby (active) side of each seal, and the seals were subjected to explosion overpressures. Both seals with the CFRP reinforcement retrofit successfully withstood explosion pressures of 60 psi or greater during the full-scale evaluations in the LLEM.

[1]Manager (Mining Engineer) – Lake Lynn Laboratory Section.
[2]Research Engineer (Mining Engineer).
Pittsburgh Research Laboratory, National Institute for Occupational Safety and Health, Pittsburgh, PA.

INTRODUCTION

Over one-half of all U.S. underground coal mines, which employ more than 70% of the U.S. underground miners, use ventilation seals to isolate the active sections of a mine from the abandoned areas. An underground explosion within the sealed area puts miners at risk when ventilation seals fail. In January 2006, the Sago Mine explosion disaster in West Virginia claimed the lives of 12 coal miners. This explosion, which was initiated within the sealed area of the mine, destroyed the mine ventilation seals that protect the miners from underground hazards. As a consequence, the Mine Safety and Health Administration (MSHA) now requires all new seal construction to withstand 50-psi or higher explosion pressures [72 Fed. Reg.[3] 28795].

There are nearly 14,000 mine seals installed in U.S. coal mines, and nearly all were designed and installed to the 20-psi standard. A priority of the National Institute for Occupational Safety and Health's (NIOSH) Pittsburgh Research Laboratory (PRL) is to investigate methods to increase the strength of existing 20-psi seals. The National Mining Association (NMA) and MSHA have identified several possible solutions that have the potential to significantly increase the pressure rating of the seals. NIOSH, MSHA, and NMA representatives met with the developer of a carbon fiber-reinforced polymer (CFRP) reinforcement technique, and NIOSH agreed to evaluate the method. The NMA, MSHA, and NIOSH then agreed on a test plan. The evaluation was conducted in NIOSH's Lake Lynn Experimental Mine (LLEM) during March-April 2007.

The CFRP reinforcement technique was designed[4] to strengthen a 20-psi-rated seal to resist the head-on explosion pressure from a methane ignition equal to 85 psi, but the seal retrofit was still only considered a 50-psi design. Designing the retrofit to withstand up to an 85-psi reflected pressure pulse generated from a head-on explosion better accounts for the variability in the strength of the existing seal, the variability in the properties and strength of the retrofit materials, and the variability in the geology of the underground coal mine strata. The CFRP reinforcement technique was first reviewed by MSHA and NIOSH for technical merit prior to conducting the LLEM evaluations. Similarly, all future seal designs and strength-enhancing retrofit designs for existing 20-psi-rated seals need to undergo a thorough review of the structural engineering design of the seal as provided by the manufacturer, including any potential health and safety issues associated with the selection and installation of the seal design materials, proper construction techniques, entry dimensions, and the anchoring and interactions to the coal mine strata at the proposed seal location. The large-scale LLEM evaluations would then complement the structural engineering designs and provide more accurate information for evaluating future seal designs and for calibrating structural design models.

This report discusses the construction techniques, testing methods, and explosion test data collected during the CFRP reinforcement seal retrofit evaluations in 2007. There are several seal reinforcement techniques that have been used in mines, including the construction of independent stronger seals in front of the existing 20-psi-rated seals or constructing a solid-concrete-block seal in front of the existing seal and then infilling the void between the seals with concrete. There are several other proposed reinforcement techniques that include the application of materials to the existing 20-psi-rated seals in a manner similar to the CFRP reinforcement technique. The CFRP reinforcement technique discussed in this report was the first such upgrade

---

[3] *Federal Register*. See Fed. Reg. in references.
[4] The fiber-reinforced construction method was designed by Ravi Kanitkar, Senior Structural Engineer, Crosby Group, Redwood City, CA.

evaluation to existing 20-psi-rated seals conducted by NIOSH in the LLEM. NIOSH does not endorse one method over another method, but reports methods that have successfully withstood the required explosion pressures.

EXPERIMENTAL MINE AND TEST PROCEDURES

Mine Explosion Tests

The full-scale explosion tests were conducted in the LLEM [Mattes et al. 1983; Triebsch and Sapko 1990]. The LLEM is part of PRL's Lake Lynn Laboratory, which is located about 50 miles southeast of Pittsburgh near Fairchance, Fayette County, PA. It is one of the world's foremost mining laboratories for conducting large-scale underground and surface safety and health research. Figure 1 shows a plan view of the LLEM.

The LLEM is a former limestone mine in which five drifts (horizontal passageways in a mine) were developed in 1979–1980 to simulate the geometries of modern U.S. coal mines. The mine has four parallel drifts: A, B, C, and D. D-drift is a 1,600-ft-long single entry that can be separated from E-drift by a movable bulkhead door. In order to simulate room-and-pillar workings, drifts A, B, and C can be used, and these drifts may be separated from E-drift by a movable bulkhead door located near the C- and E-drift intersection (Figure 1). The A-, B- and C-drifts are each approximately 1,600 ft long, with seven crosscuts at the inby end. C- and D-drifts are connected by E-drift, a 500-ft-long entry that simulates a longwall face.

The explosion tests were conducted in the C-drift entry area. The entry and crosscuts are approximately 20 ft wide by about 6½ ft high, with cross-sectional areas of 130–140 ft^2. Figure 2 is a closeup plan view of the seal test area in the multiple-entry area of the LLEM. In this example, there are seals in the first four crosscuts from the face or closed end of C-drift. Note that, at the LLEM, the first crosscut is the one nearest the face (closed end). The flammable natural gas-air volume (ignition zone) is limited to the 47-ft-long butt entry located inby crosscut 1 in C-drift. The ignition zone is contained by a plastic diaphragm attached to a wooden perimeter framework near the outby end of the 47-ft-long butt entry. The bulkhead door is closed between C-drift and E-drift before the test.

For an explosion test, the natural gas was injected into the ignition zone, and an electric fan with an explosion-proof motor housing was used to mix the natural gas with the air in the ignition zone. Sample lines within the ignition zone were used to draw samples to an infrared analyzer for continuous monitoring of the methane concentrations. The flammable natural gas-air volume was ignited using a triple-point ignition source. This ignition source consists of three sets of two 100-J electric matches that are equally spaced at midheight across the closed end (face) and ignited at the same time. The resultant explosion pressure travels out C-drift. Figure 2 represents the unconfined, side-on explosion pressure loading method that was requested by MSHA for use in evaluating the strength of seal designs within the LLEM from 1990 through 2005 [Stephan 1990a,b; Greninger et al. 1991; Weiss et al. 1993a,b,c; 1996; 1997; 1999; 2002].

The ignition of the approximately 10% methane-in-air concentration within the 47-ft-long butt entry of C-drift typically generated unconfined, side-on explosion pressures at the crosscut seal locations ranging from approximately 20 to 25 psi at the various seal locations. Typically, shelves of pulverized coal dust located outby the gas zone would be added to generate higher side-on explosion pressures against the seals, although this increased side-on explosion pressure loading could have also been accomplished by expanding the volume of the gas zone. Igniting increasingly larger volumes of flammable methane-air will result in increasingly higher explosion pressures, although this is dependent on other factors such as the location of the ignition source within the flammable volume [Sapko et al. 1987; Zipf et al. 2007].

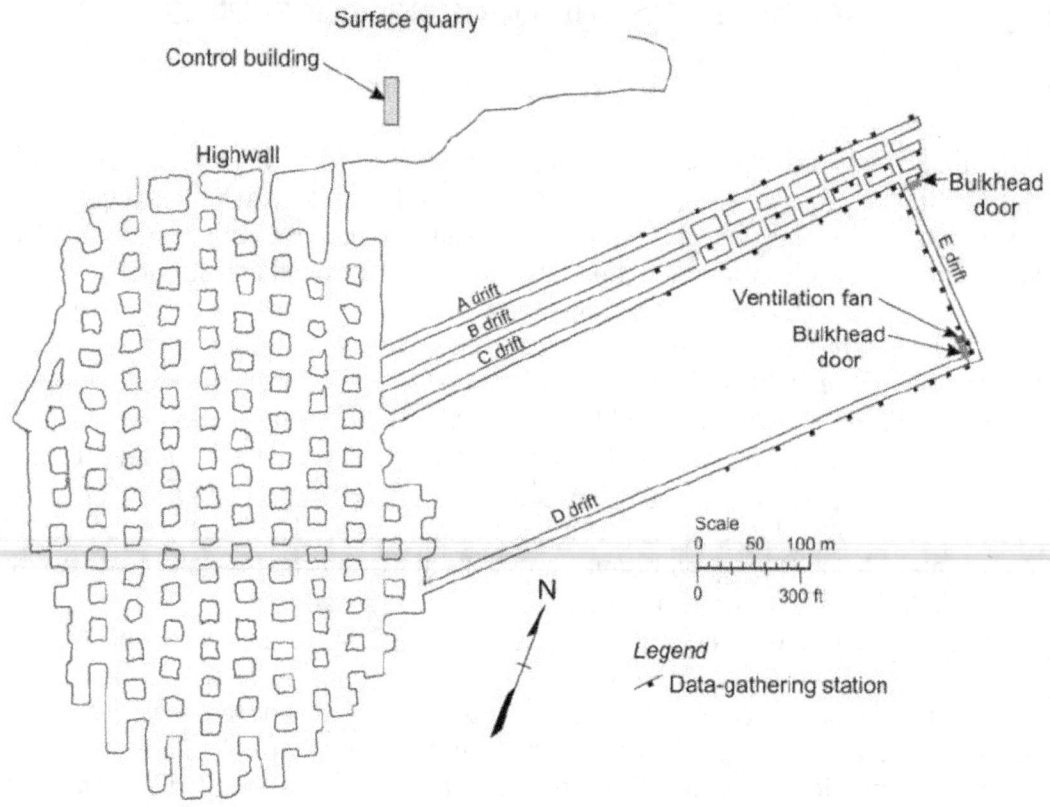

Figure 1.—Plan view of the Lake Lynn Experimental Mine (LLEM).

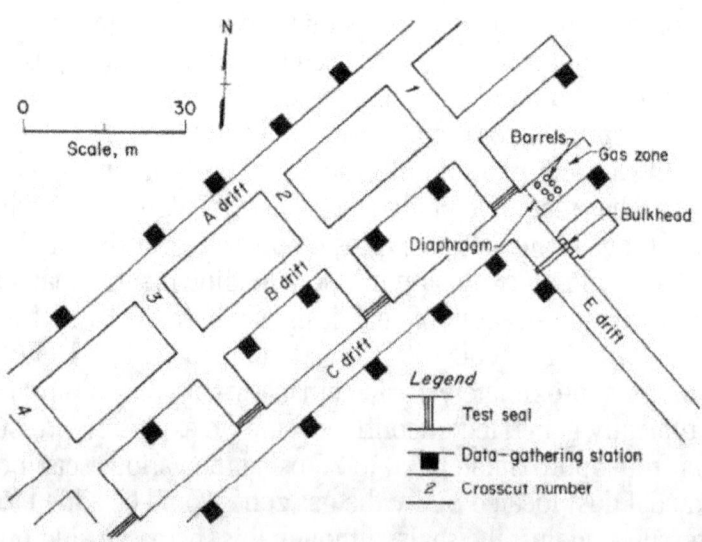

Figure 2.—Seal test area in the LLEM.

The 1992 revisions to the 30 CFR[5] 75.335 sealing regulations were based on the general consensus that explosions were most likely to originate from the active working sections, and any subsequent explosion pressures acting on the seals would be more representative of a side-on loading that would not exceed 20 psi. Based on the conclusions of the MSHA mine explosion investigation reports in the 1990s and early 2000s, any seals that were destroyed and/or damaged due to explosions that originated from within the sealed areas were primarily a result of inadequate seal construction due to poor quality-control issues, and the explosion pressures were estimated to be less than 20 psi. Since the Sago Mine disaster in 2006 and the subsequent MSHA investigation [Gates et al. 2007], MSHA has issued new seal strength requirements, and the NIOSH evaluations within the LLEM are now focused on the effects of a confined, head-on explosion pressure on seal performance.

During the evaluation of the CFRP reinforcement technique, one retrofitted alternative 20-psi-rated seal was evaluated using a confined, head-on (or face-on) explosion pressure loading method. A second retrofitted alternative seal was constructed in an open crosscut and thereby subjected to a confined, side-on explosion pressure loading (a sweeping pressure pulse). Two seals from previous evaluations remained in crosscuts 1 and 2 between B- and C-drifts, and they served to block those open crosscuts. One of the retrofitted alternative seals was installed across C-drift between crosscuts 3 and 4 to accomplish the desired confined, head-on explosion pressure loading method. The second retrofitted alternative seal was installed in crosscut 3 and subjected to a confined side-on explosion pressure loading. This confined head-on evaluation method will be further discussed in the "Explosion Test Results" section later in this report.

Instrumentation

Each LLEM drift has 10 data-gathering (DG) stations inset in the rib wall at the locations shown in Figures 1–2. Each DG station houses a strain gauge transducer to measure the explosion pressure and an optical sensor to detect the flame arrival. The explosion pressure is dynamic in nature and has two components: an omnidirectional pressure component (the pressure that is exerted in all directions and is measured perpendicular to the gas flow) and a wind or velocity pressure component (pressure due to gas flow). The total explosion pressure is the sum of the omnidirectional pressure and the wind or velocity pressure. The transducers in the DG stations in the wall measure the omnidirectional pressure. All of the explosion pressures reported in this publication are overpressures or gauge pressures (pressures above local atmospheric pressure) rather than absolute pressures.

Nagy [1981, p. 58] referred to the omnidirectional pressure as the "static pressure" to differentiate it from the "dynamic pressure," or velocity component. However, the omnidirectional pressure is not actually "static" as it does vary with time during the explosion. This terminology by Nagy had been used in previous U.S. Bureau of Mines and NIOSH reports, but it was confusing to many readers and will no longer be used.

The pressure transducers of particular interest for these seal evaluations were installed along the C-drift rib at 234, 304, and 403 ft from the face at the DG station positions shown in Figures 1–2. The pressure data collected in all of the DG stations in B- and C-drifts are listed in the Appendix (Tables A–1 and A–2). There were also pressure transducers mounted on the inby side of the seal that was installed across C-drift and on the C-drift side of the seals in the

---

[5] *Code of Federal Regulations.* See CFR in references.

crosscuts. One or two of the transducers faced the explosion forces and measured the total explosion pressures at the seals. Other transducers were oriented perpendicular to the oncoming explosion and measured the omnidirectional pressure. The velocity (or wind) pressure would act on objects in an open entry as the explosion travels down the entry. When the velocity (or wind) pressure reaches a solid surface, such as a seal across the entry or crosscut, the velocity would go to zero, and the total explosion pressure would be approximately the same as the omnidirectional pressure at that location. In addition, when the pressure pulse reaches a seal, it is reflected, and the resulting total reflected pressure can be about twice the incoming pressure pulse value.

Figure 3 shows the heavy steel housings and mounts for the pressure transducers on the explosion (or C-drift) side of the low-density block seal in crosscut 3. Similar housing and mounts are used at the other seal locations. For these tests (LLEM tests 508–509) involving the CFRP reinforcement technique for upgrading the strength of seals, there were pressure transducers placed in front of each of the two candidate seals. For the 24-in-thick, low-density block seal in crosscut 3, two transducers were mounted horizontally to face the incoming pressure wave—one mounted within a steel housing on a steel post anchored near the center of the seal and one embedded flush into the seal near the center. The crosscut 3 seal also had one transducer mounted vertically on both the inby and outby crosscut ribs. A vertically mounted transducer on the center post was not used in crosscut 3 during these evaluations (although the housing on the steel post is shown in Figure 3). The original intent of the transducers mounted vertically on both the inby and outby crosscut ribs was to document the pressures exerted on the seal as a function of time to better understand the nonuniform pressure loading (a sweeping pulse) on a crosscut seal. However, it must be noted that the peak pressures recorded on these transducers were significantly influenced by the reflected and/or focused pressure pulses occurring at these locations. When the original outward traveling explosion pressure pulse interacted with the crosscut seal, the transducer located on the outby seal-rib interface measured a higher pressure compared to the transducers located at the center of the seal and the inby seal-rib interface. A similar situation was experienced at the transducer located on the inby seal-rib interface when the inwardly traveling reflected pressure pulse (resulting when the head-on explosion encountered the seal across C-drift) passed the crosscut seal.

For the 4-ft-thick pumpable cementitious foam seal across C-drift, two transducers were mounted horizontally to face the incoming (head-on) pressure wave—one mounted to a steel post anchored near the center of the seal and one embedded flush into the seal near the center. The seal across C-drift also had two transducers mounted perpendicular to the gas flow—one mounted vertically to the steel post anchored near the center of the seal and one mounted on the left outby rib next to the seal.

Other instruments may also be installed at various locations in the LLEM during an explosion test. Behind each seal were linear variable displacement transducers[6] (LVDTs), as shown in Figure 4. The LVDT measures the movement of the seal during an explosion [Weiss et al. 1999, pp. 5–6]. An LVDT was mounted midheight and midwidth on the outby face (nonexplosion side) of each seal. For the crosscut 3 seal, LVDTs were also mounted midheight and one-quarter distance from each rib. For the seal across C-drift, an additional LVDT was mounted midheight and one-quarter distance from the right inby rib. Also shown in Figure 4 are the horizontal and vertical breakwires used to measure the approximate time of seal failure.

---

[6] Also referred to as "linear variable differential transformers."

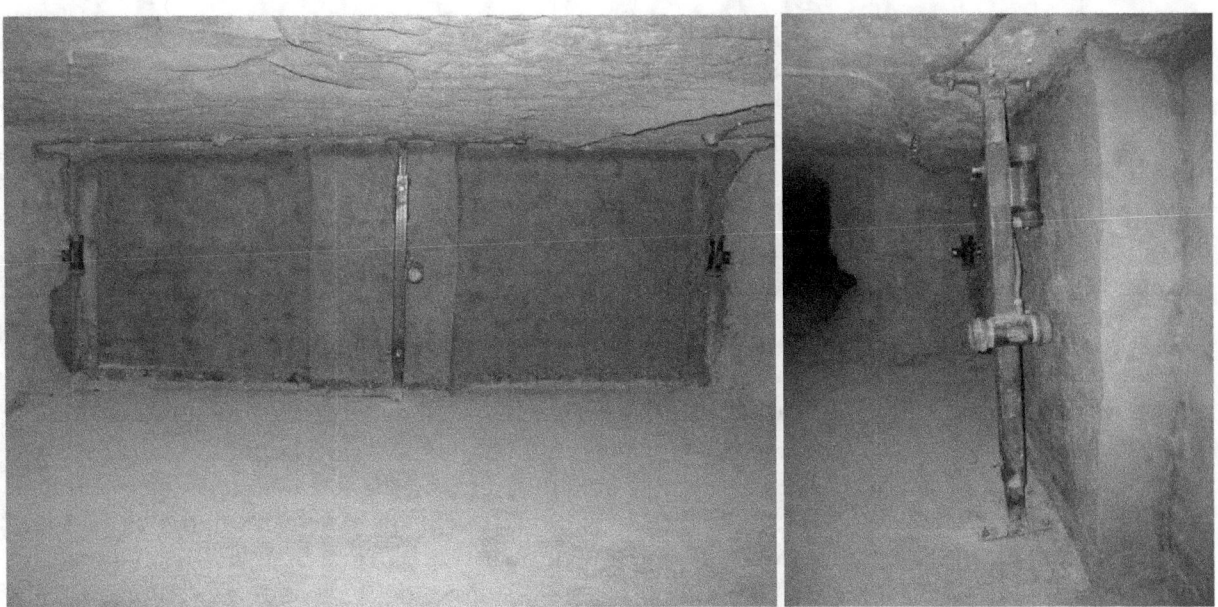

Figure 3.—Front view *(left)* and side view *(right)* of housings and mounts for the pressure transducers on the explosion (or C-drift) side of the low-density block seal in crosscut 3.

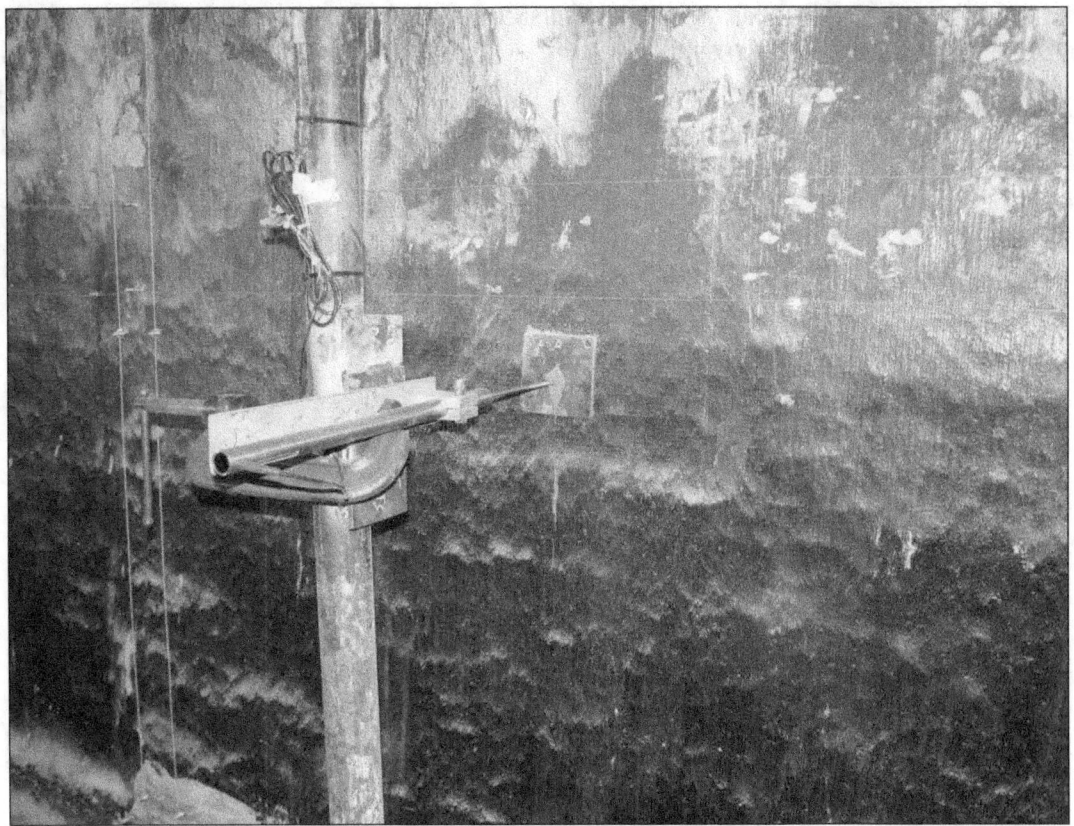

Figure 4.—LVDT mounted behind seal to measure movement of the seal during an explosion. The vertical yellow wires to the left of the sensor post and the horizontal blue wires above the LVDT anchoring plate on the seal are the breakwires.

During the explosion tests, a high-speed, PC-based National Instruments Corp. data acquisition system collected the data from the various instruments at a sampling rate of 1,500 samples per second. The reported data were smoothed (or averaged) over 15 points, or 10 ms. A second Kinetic Systems, Inc., data acquisition system collected the data at a sampling rate of 5,000 samples per second (51-point smoothing). The data are smoothed to eliminate the high spike transient noise signals, but smoothing can reduce the real pressure data and thereby reduce the maximum reported peak pressure. However, the raw, unsmoothed data are also analyzed for the pressure transducers of particular importance.

Air Leakage Determinations

Measurements of the air leakages through the seals were taken before and after each of the explosion tests. To measure the leakage through the seal, the bulkhead door at D-drift is first closed to allow for the pressurizing of the entry area inby the C-drift seal locations. The volume inby the seals is pressurized by operating the fan at the different speed settings in the blowing mode (pushing air into the mine). Since the airflow in C-drift is blocked by the seals and the D-drift bulkhead door is closed, the pressure differential across the seals increases for each of the four fan settings. Typically, the pressure differential across the seals ranges from 0.8 in H_2O at the lowest fan setting to upwards of 4.5 in H_2O at the highest (fourth) fan setting. A copper tube, with a pressure gauge on the outby side of the seal, extends through each seal as a means to measure this pressure differential. A relatively airtight wood framework with a brattice curtain overlay is installed on the outby (nonexplosion) side of each seal. A circular hole, the size of the anemometer, is cut in the brattice curtain to measure the air leakage through the seal at the varying pressure differentials across the seal (Figure 5). For additional details on the air leakage measurement technique used during the LLEM evaluations, refer to Weiss et al. [2002, pp. 6–7].

A seal must exhibit minimal air leakage rates before and after each explosion test, and these rates must meet the MSHA-established guidelines for seal evaluations within the LLEM. For pressure differentials up to 1 in H_2O, air leakage must not exceed 100 cfm. For pressure differentials greater than 3 in H_2O, air leakage must be less than 250 cfm.

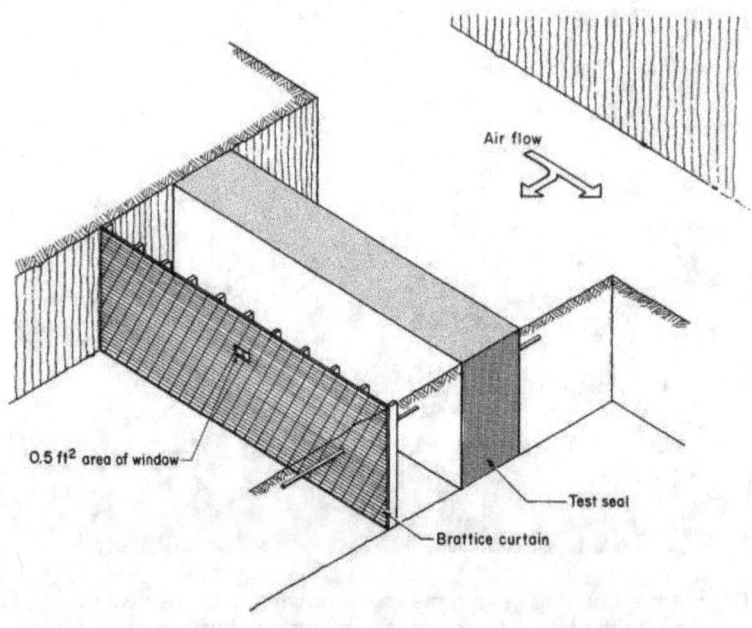

Air flow

0.5 ft^2 area of window

Test seal

Brattice curtain

Figure 5.—Schematic of setup for seal leakage test.

SEAL CONSTRUCTION

Seals installed from a previous evaluation program in 2006 were left in place in crosscuts 1 and 2. The seal in crosscut 1 was a 16-in-thick, solid-concrete-block seal with a 16-in by 32-in interlocked center pilaster and simulated keying (hitching) to the ribs and floor. The seal in crosscut 2 was a 40-in-thick, low-density block seal without rib and floor keying (unhitched). Both of these seals were subjected to seven previous explosion tests. To ensure that the crosscut 2 seal did not fail during this current evaluation, 6-in by 6-in by ½-in thick steel angle (American Society for Testing and Materials (ASTM) A–36) was installed on the B-drift (nonexplosion) side of the seal across the roof and floor to buttress the seal. The angle was secured to the concrete floor and limestone roof using 1-in-diam, 9- and 12-in-long anchor bolts (Kwik Bolt III manufactured by Hilti Inc., Tulsa, OK) on less than 18-in centers. A vertical center angle was also secured in place behind the seal. All gaps between the steel angle and roof and the steel angle and seal were filled with high-strength mortar (BlocBond, product No. 1225–51, a fiber-reinforced surface bonding cement manufactured by Quikrete Co., Atlanta, GA; 50-lb average weight per bag). The candidate seals for evaluating the CFRP reinforcement technique were constructed in crosscut 3 and across C-drift between crosscuts 3 and 4 at a location 320 ft from the closed end (C–320).

Cementitious Pumpable Foam Seal

A 48-in-thick pumpable cementitious foam seal using material with a designed 150-psi average compressive strength at 28 days was installed across C-drift at a distance of 320 ft from the closed-end ignition zone (location "C–320") (see Figure 2). The purpose of placing a seal using a material with a lower average compressive strength than normal was to account for the variability and potential quality-control issues that can be associated with the construction of all types of pumpable cementitious foam seals in mines. To be conservative, MSHA wanted the seal retrofit to be conducted on a structure that was representative of a lower-strength seal. The seal manufacturer was requested to place a seal with an approximate average compressive strength equal to 150 psi. The seal was constructed by personnel from the R. G. Johnson Co., Washington, PA. These types of seal designs (although using materials with higher compressive strengths) were originally evaluated against the unconfined, side-on explosion overpressures in the early 1990s [Greninger et al. 1991; Weiss et al. 1993a; 1996] and represent flat-wall designs. Additionally, the seal design for this evaluation was constructed of material such that its overall strength would minimally survive the previous 20 psi-level explosion overpressure requirement. The pumpable cementitious foam seal is a plug-type seal; this seal is not keyed into the ribs or floor. The average dimensions in C-drift at the seal location are 18.7 ft wide by 7.3 ft high. The seal was constructed on the 8-in-thick reinforced concrete floor in C-drift.

The inby and outby form walls each consisted of six 6-in by 4-in untreated hardwood posts cut to various lengths to fit the entry height (Figure 6). A post was positioned approximately 8 in from each rib with an approximately 42-in center-to-center spacing between each post across the entry. Wood wedges were used between the top of each post and the mine roof to tighten each post. The inby and outby form walls were spaced to provide an interior seal thickness of 48 in. Rough-cut hardwood boards (8 in wide by 1 in thick) were attached with nails to the interior side of the vertical wood posts on each form wall. The spacing between these horizontal crossboards was approximately 8 in. The boards were installed as close as possible against the roof, floor, and ribs. Brattice cloth ("Dura-Skrim" manufactured by Raven Industries, Inc., Sioux Falls, SD, MSHA approval No. 07–BA040001–0) was then attached to the interior of each form wall, overlapping approximately 4 in on the roof and ribs. Flexible metal straps (1 in wide) were attached to the roof, ribs, and posts to secure the overlapped brattice cloth in place and minimize leakage of the cementitious slurry during pumping (Figure 7). The completed form wall is shown in Figure 6. Eye bolts were attached to the inside of each vertical post at three heights (approximately one-quarter, one-half, and three-quarter heights). A ⅛-in-diam galvanized steel cable (seven-strand cable with seven wires per strand) was secured to the eye bolts on the opposing vertical posts on the inby and outby form walls (Figure 7). These cables serve as form ties and prevent the outward displacement of the form walls during the pumping of the cementitious slurry. There were six rows of cable ties across the entry (one cable for each inby/outby post set) between the form walls at each of the three heights. Fiberglass insulation was used along the ribs and floor to minimize cementitious slurry leakage between the brattice cloth liner and strata. Additionally, polyurethane foam (Hilti CF810 Crack & Joint Pro Foam manufactured by Hilti, Inc., Tulsa, OK) was applied at the roof of the inby form wall to minimize leakages during the slurry injection process. Construction of the form walls required 2½ days to complete, with three miners working 8-hr shifts, or 60 worker-hours.

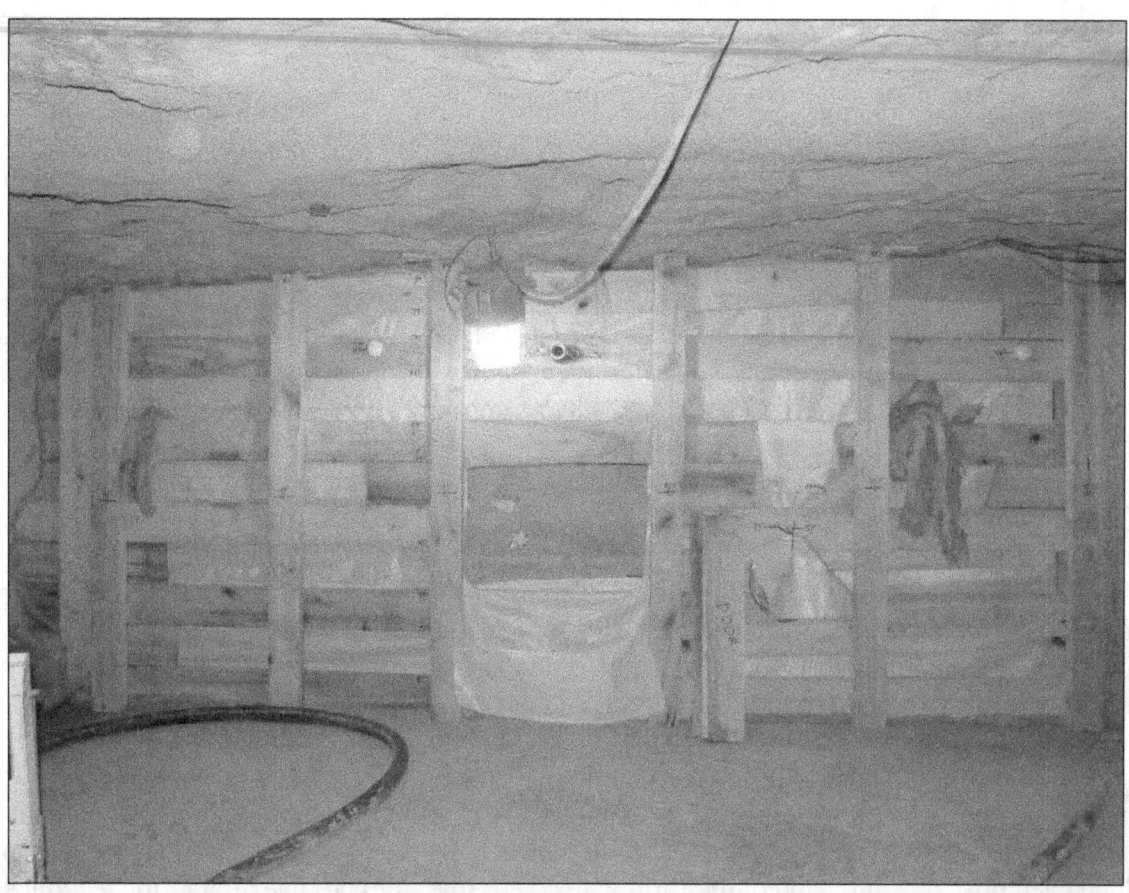

Figure 6.—Outby form wall for the pumpable cementitious foam seal.

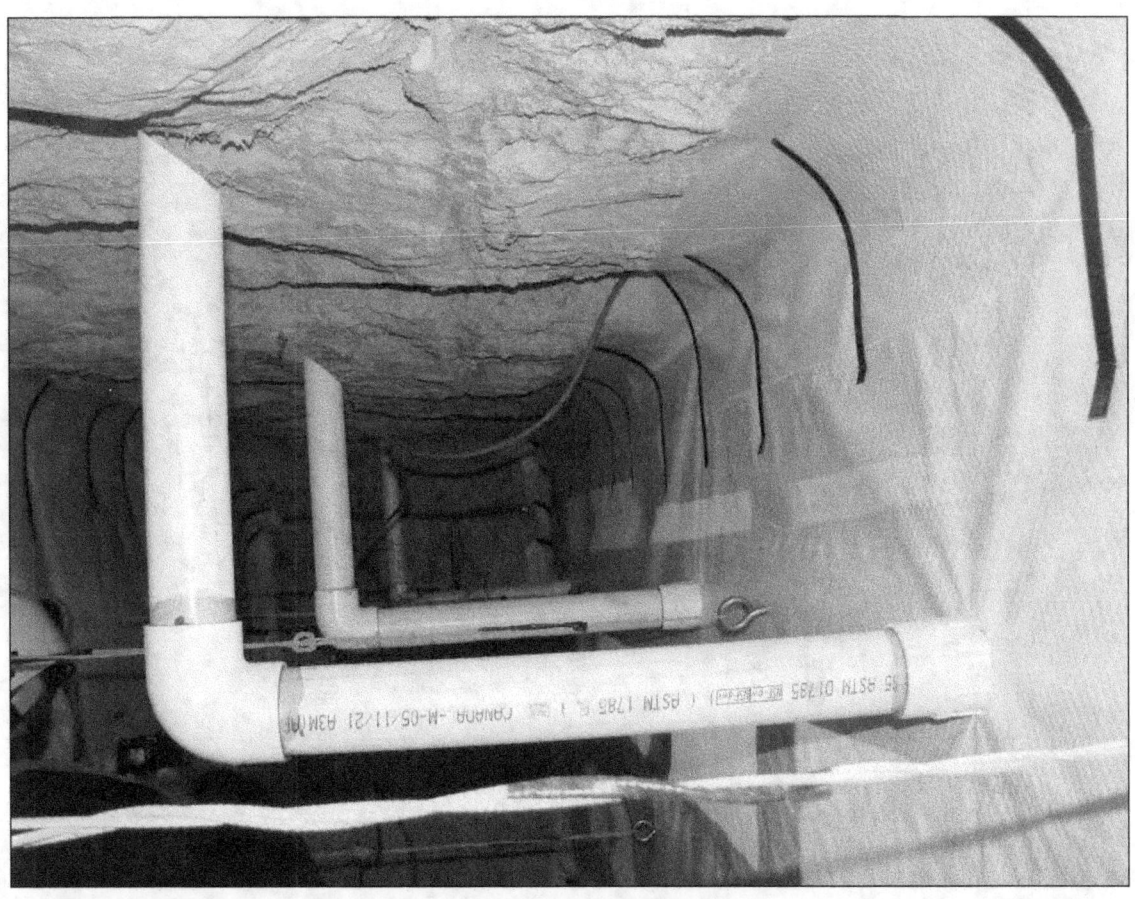

Figure 7.—View between the two form walls showing the injection and bleeder pipes, the flexible metal straps holding the overlapped brattice tight to the strata, and the steel cable ties between the inby and outby form wall posts.

The center opening in the outby form wall (Figure 6) is initially used to pump the slurry between the form walls. As the slurry height increases between the form walls, brattice cloth and crossboards are used to incrementally close and seal the center opening. The slurry injection for the top third of the seal is accomplished through a center injection port (Figure 6). Bleeder pipes are used as an indicator as to when the slurry has reached the mine roof. The injection port and bleeder pipes are installed through one of the upper crossboards. Internal pipes connected to the injection port and bleeder pipes are installed to the highest roof points between the two form walls to ensure complete filling of the cementitious slurry to the mine roof (Figure 7). The bleeders are capped during the pumping operation when the slurry begins to flow through the bleeder pipes. A 200-gal tank, containing a mixture of 120 gal of water and 5 gal of foam concentrate, was pressurized to 65–80 psi. Cement (Saylor's Type I portland cement manufactured by Essroc Cement Corp., Nazareth, PA) was loaded into an electric-powered screw auger and mixed with the water and foam mixture (Figure 8). The slurry mixture was then pumped between the form walls (Figure 9). The weight of a bucket filled with the cementitious foam slurry was used to calculate the density of the slurry (Figure 10). Based on this calculated density, the feed rates of the cement auger and the water/foam mixture could then be adjusted to provide the desired density for the slurry that would then be pumped between the form walls.

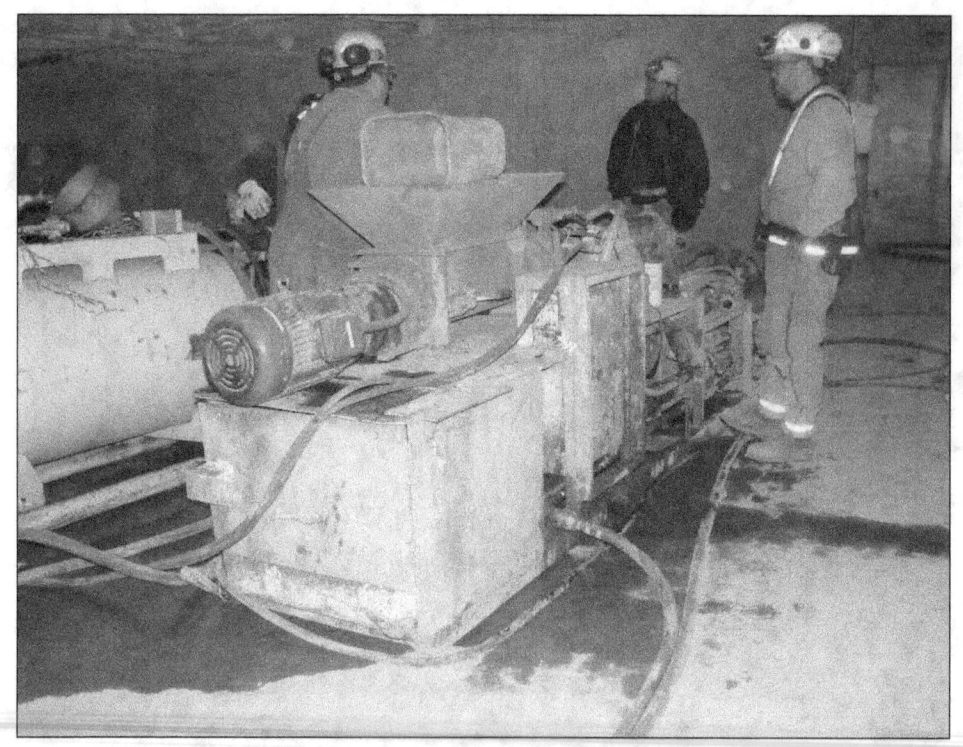

Figure 8.—Electric-powered screw auger *(center of photo)* for the cement feed and the heated water and foam tank *(left side of photo)*.

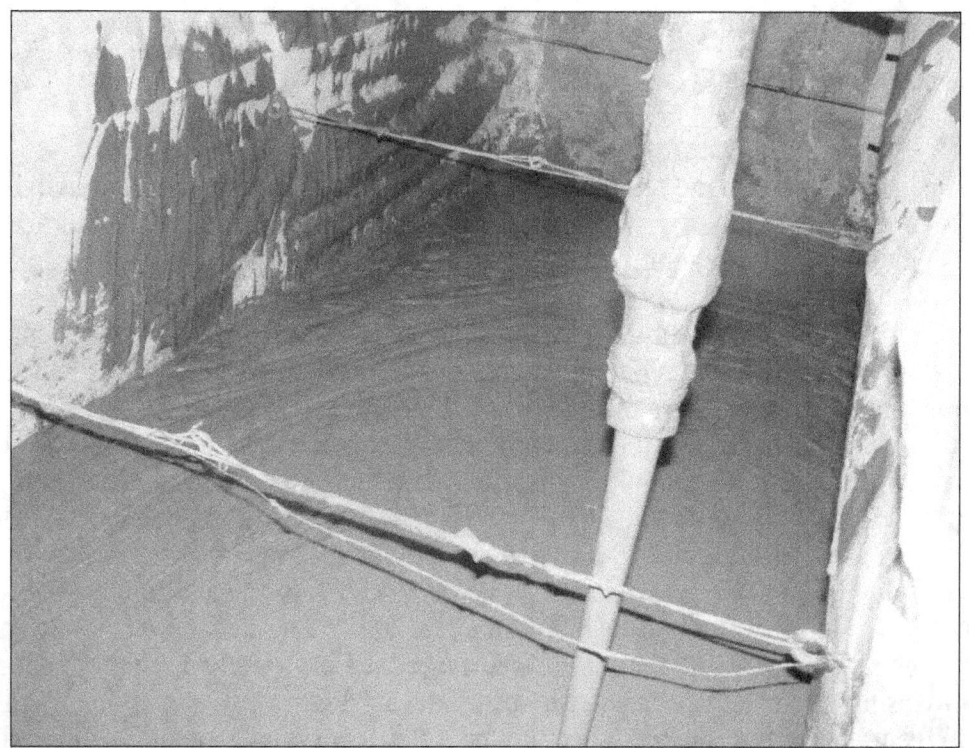

Figure 9.—Pumping of cementitious foam slurry between form walls.

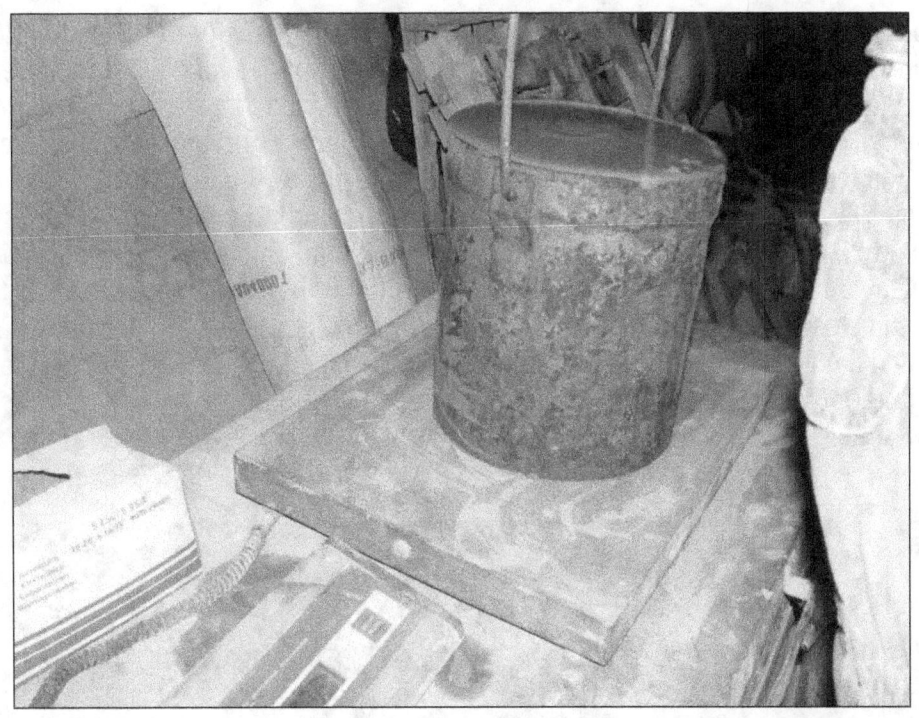

Figure 10.—Digital scale and bucket used to calculate the density of the cementitious foam slurry.

The first attempt of constructing the seal with a lower-than-usual density cementitious foam slurry material (150-psi average) resulted in the collapse of the foam structure at some point after the first-day pour and before the second-day pour. Several reasons can explain this seal collapse. The average compressive strength of the material was significantly lower than requested for this seal. During the slurry-filling process, the material compressive strength is based on the weight of the material samples taken before and during the pours. The unit weight bucket used to hold the sample and the electronic scales used to weigh the bucket samples were rarely cleaned of the waste material that flowed over the bucket and/or spilled onto the scales. The extra weight of the sample material may have adversely affected the calculated unit weight of the sample and the subsequent adjustments made to the mix. The cold mine water used for the mix water may have affected the initial set time for the material. A significant amount of bleed water was also observed on the concrete floor of the LLEM during the slurry-filling process. Bleed water will migrate downward toward the mine floor since the aerated material is less dense than the bleed water. This may have resulted in voids formed within the central portion of the seal at or near the floor. Samples obtained from the seal placements revealed that voids formed at the bottom of the sample containers since the aerated concrete will tend to float on the bleed water. For the material placement within the seal, more bleed water would accumulate in the central portion of the seal since this is the location where the seal material was discharged from the hose. The voids forming within or at the bottom of the seal in combination with a slow set time (due to the cold mine water), low material strength, and an excessively high first pour with the lower-strength material are plausible explanations for why the central portion of the seal collapsed. After the collapse, the outby form wall was disassembled and the first-day pour material was removed. The outby form wall was then rebuilt.

13

During the second attempt of constructing the seal, the density of the cementitious foam slurry material was slightly increased (with the goal still being to achieve a final cured material with <200-psi average compressive strength), the height of each day's pour was significantly reduced to prevent the material collapse, and the mine water was preheated (the heated water temperature ranged from 66 °F to 84 °F, with an average of 75 °F based on periodic readings of the outlet water temperature gauge). On day 1, a 38-min pumping time resulted in a slurry height of 31 in. On day 2, a 71-min pumping time increased the total slurry height to 68 in between the form walls. Day 3 required a 32-min pumping time through the center injection port (Figure 11) to complete the closure to the mine roof. Twice during this final injection period, the slurry was forced between the form walls under pressure to ensure that all of the voids were filled. The slurry-pumping operations required three miners a total of ~2.3 hr (or 7 worker-hours) to complete the seal.

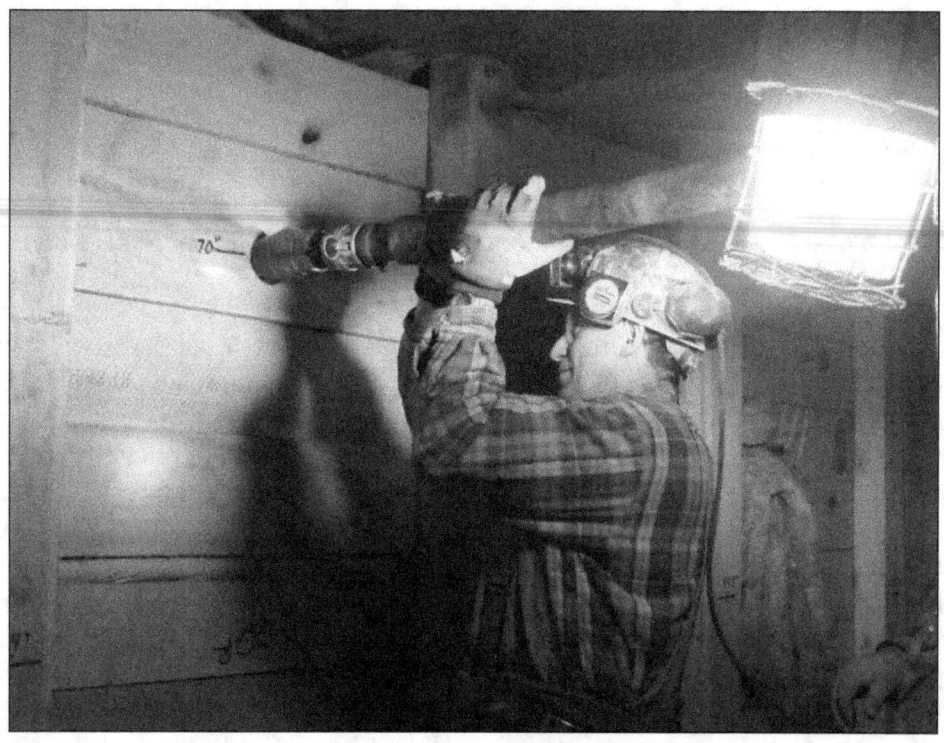

Figure 11.—Connection of the slurry injection hose for filling the top third of the seal.

Samples of the cementitious foam slurry for the second seal were randomly taken during the pumping operations by R. G. Johnson Co., Inc. (tested by Professional Service Industries, Inc., Pittsburgh, PA) and Transco Products, Inc., Chicago, IL (tested by Construction Technology Laboratories, Skokie, IL). The samples collected by R. G. Johnson were contained in Styrofoam four-cylinder sample packs (capped with a Styrofoam lid) and averaged 143-psi compressive strength (individual sample results ranged from 100 to 190 psi) after an average 36-day cure period. The samples collected by Transco Products were contained in individual airtight and watertight capped plastic sample containers and averaged 241-psi compressive strength (individual sample results ranged from 190 to 290 psi) after an average 41-day cure period. The collected samples and compressive strength tests for both sets of samples did not meet all of the ASTM testing standards, which may account for the differences in the test results. Also, the additional handling[7] of the Transco Products samples may have reduced the air content in the samples, resulting in higher compressive strengths. The differences between the required strength and the actual strength further demonstrates the potential quality-control issues with continuous-feed volume batching of the cementitious foam material in controlling the slurry mix and strength of the material.

To document the heat release during the cementitious foam curing process, a series of thermocouples were installed between the form walls at one-fourth, one-half, and three-quarter height near the center of the seal. Figure 12 is a graph showing the results of internal temperature measurements every 5 min during the initial 7-day cure period for the cementitious foam seal. Within the first approximately 10 hr of cure time for each of the three cementitious foam slurry pours, the internal temperatures as measured by the thermocouples increased to a high temperature ranging between 88 and 98 °C (190 and 208 °F). After this initial 10-hr cure time, the internal temperatures of the curing cementitious foam material steadily decreased over time. Seven days after the first pour, the temperatures on all three thermocouples ranged between 40 and 50 °C (104 and 122 °F), while 21 days after the first pour, the temperatures on all three thermocouples were ~18 °C (~64 °F).

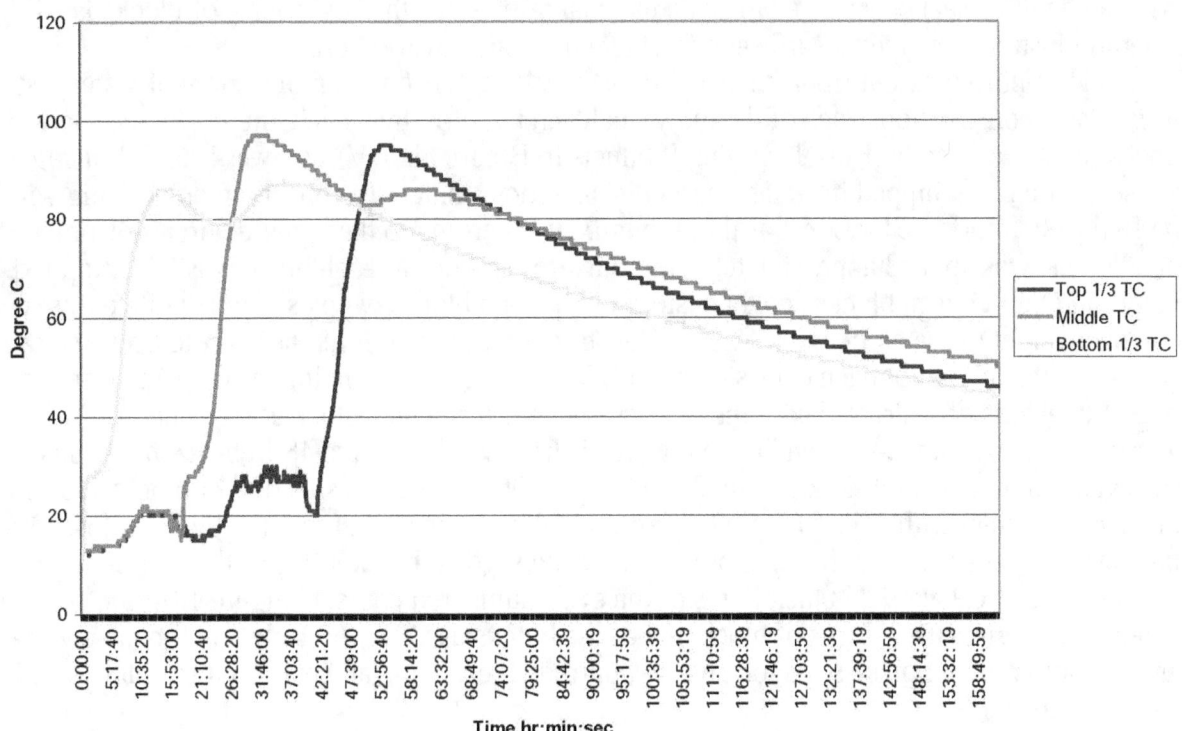

Figure 12.—Temperature measurements during the initial 7-day cure period for the pumpable cementitious foam seal at C–320. (TC = thermocouple.)

---

[7]The slurry material was transferred from the bucket into a plastic bag, the plastic sample molds were filled from the bag, then the samples were agitated with a rod.

Low-Density Block Seal

A 24-in-thick, low-density block seal with a 48-in by 48-in center pilaster and simulated keying of the ribs and floor (using the 6-in steel angle) was installed in crosscut 3 between B- and C-drifts of the LLEM (Figure 2). This seal design was originally evaluated against unconfined, side-on explosion overpressures during LLEM evaluations in 1994 [Weiss et al. 1996] and represents the 20-psi pilaster-type alternate seals used in coal mines. The average dimensions in crosscut 3 at the seal location are 18.8 ft wide by 6.75 ft high.

The seal was constructed approximately 6–7 ft into the crosscut (as measured from the C-drift side) on a small concrete foundation (leveling pad) that tapered from 0- to 4-in thick (as measured from C- to B-drifts) on top of an 8-in-thick reinforced concrete floor. The roof and floor slope in crosscut 3 is approximately 6% as measured from C-drift to B-drift and approximately 5% rib to rib. This pad is leveled only along the C- to B-drift plane to provide a level surface for the first course of block. As a result, the use of the leveling pad could affect the angle of interface between the top of the seal and the mine roof, which may provide a means for the sloping mine roof to confine and resist seal movement (to an unknown degree) at the roof-seal interface during the explosion tests that originate in C-drift compared to any resistance obtained had the seal been constructed within a level entry or an entry that sloped in the opposite direction (where the roof would "open up" in the direction that the seal would displace). Similar issues are associated with a seal constructed in an actual coal mine since the first course of blocks is still generally installed on a level surface to facilitate the wall construction.

The entire crosscut (roof, ribs, and floor) was dampened with a fine spray of water just prior to seal construction. Each of the individual 8-in by 16-in by 24-in Omega 384 low-density blocks (manufactured by Burrell Mining Products in Bluefield, WV) was wet-brushed (using a coarse bristle brush dipped in water) to remove any loose material to ensure good bonding with the BlocBond mortar. BlocBond, as properly mixed according to the manufacturer's recommendations, was applied approximately ¼ in thick to the floor as each block was laid. Approximately 127 full Omega blocks and 44 custom-cut Omega blocks were used to complete this seal. Average weight of the blocks was 45.7 lb. Construction of the odd-numbered courses (first, third, fifth, seventh, and ninth) each consisted of ~17 Omega blocks (16-in dimension parallel to the longitudinal axis of C-drift). Six of these blocks were offset a half-block at the center of the crosscut (three toward C-drift and three toward B-drift) to provide the 48-in by 48-in pilaster. The even-numbered courses (2nd, 4th, 6th, 8th, and 10th) each consisted of ~14 blocks (16-in dimension parallel with C-drift), with four additional blocks each cut to 12 in by 24 in (used for the pilaster extensions on either side of the seal). The vertical block joints of the odd-numbered courses offset those vertical block joints of the even-numbered courses (Figure 13). The completed seal required 10 courses of block. All of the blocks used for the 10th (final) course were cut and mortared into place so as to leave an approximately 2-in gap between these blocks and the mine roof.

Figure 14 illustrates the alternating courses and staggered block joints. The construction techniques for this seal included staggering the vertical block joints a minimum of 4 in (one-quarter the length of the block), maintaining at least a ¼-in BlocBond mortar joint (block-to-block interfaces and block-to-strata interfaces, including the floor and ribs) and providing a ¼-in coating of BlocBond on both faces (sides) of the seal. Approximately 56 bags of properly mixed BlocBond were used as joint mortar and sealant. To tighten the seal with wood wedges at the mine roof without damaging the Omega block, one layer of 12-in-wide by 1-in-thick hardwood planks was run lengthwise (rib to rib) from each side of the seal on the top course of block of the main seal wall (Figure 15) and on the 12-in by 48-in pilaster extension on each side of the seal. The plank joints were staggered between the front and back planks. The planking was set in a thin layer of BlocBond. From each side of the seal, wood wedges were then driven perpendicular to these planks between the mine roof and planks as a means to tighten the entire seal structure. The wedges were driven on 6- to 12-in centers (Figure 16). The main wall planking was positioned and wedged first, then the two cut blocks used for the top course pilaster extension were mortared into place on each side of the seal. After these blocks were installed, a 12-in-long by 48-in-long wood plank was positioned and wedged over this pilaster extension on each side of the seal. BlocBond was then used to completely fill all remaining gaps between the wedges and mine roof.

Lengths of 6-in by 6-in by ½-in thick steel angle (ASTM A–36) were then installed on each rib and along the floor (against the main seal wall and the pilaster) on both sides of the seal. The steel angle was secured to the ribs and floor using 1-in-diam by 9-in (or 12-in) long anchor bolts (Hilti Kwik Bolt III). The maximum bolt spacing was 18 in. All gaps between the steel angle and ribs and the steel angle and seal were filled with BlocBond. Figure 17 shows the completed 24-in-thick, low-density block seal in crosscut 3 as seen from the C-drift (explosion) side. Seal construction required approximately 9 hr (or 36 worker-hours) to complete. This did not include the time required to mobilize the construction equipment and materials at the site.

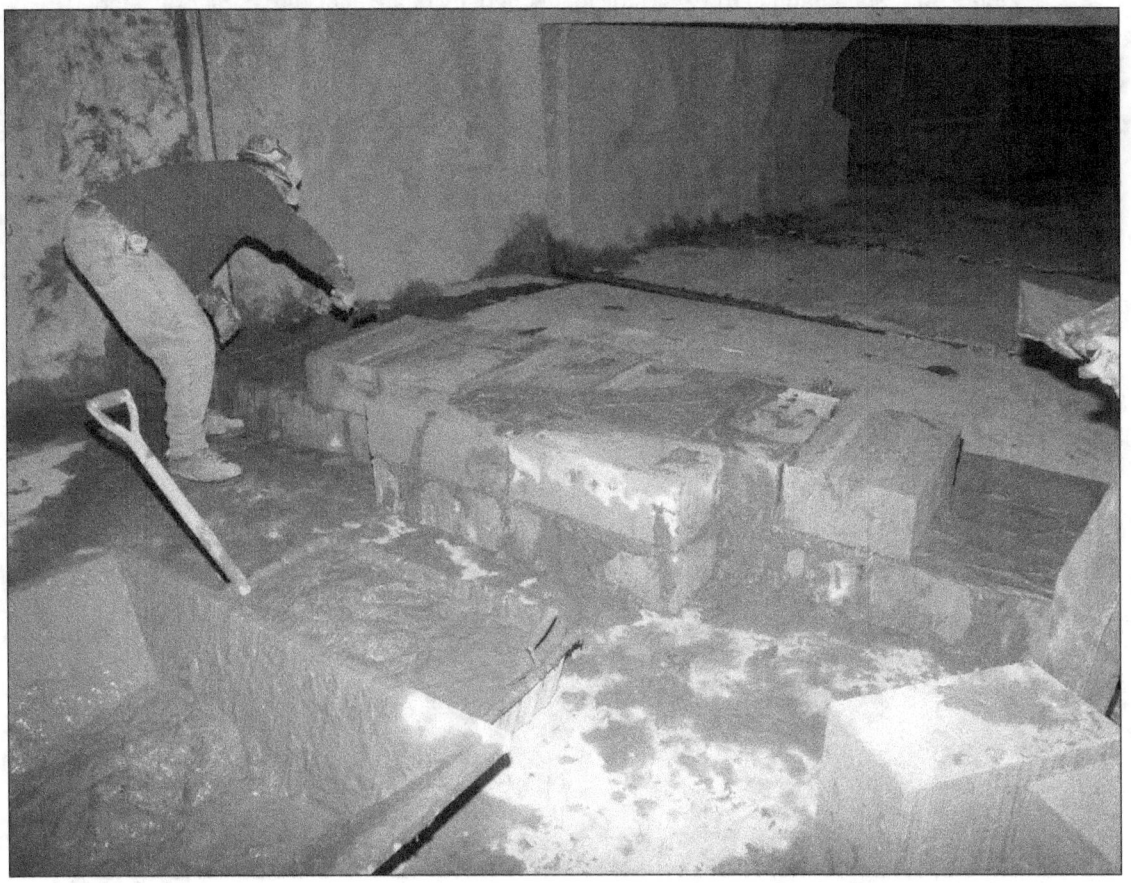

Figure 13.—Full wet-bed construction on all horizontal and vertical block joints. The vertical block joints are staggered.

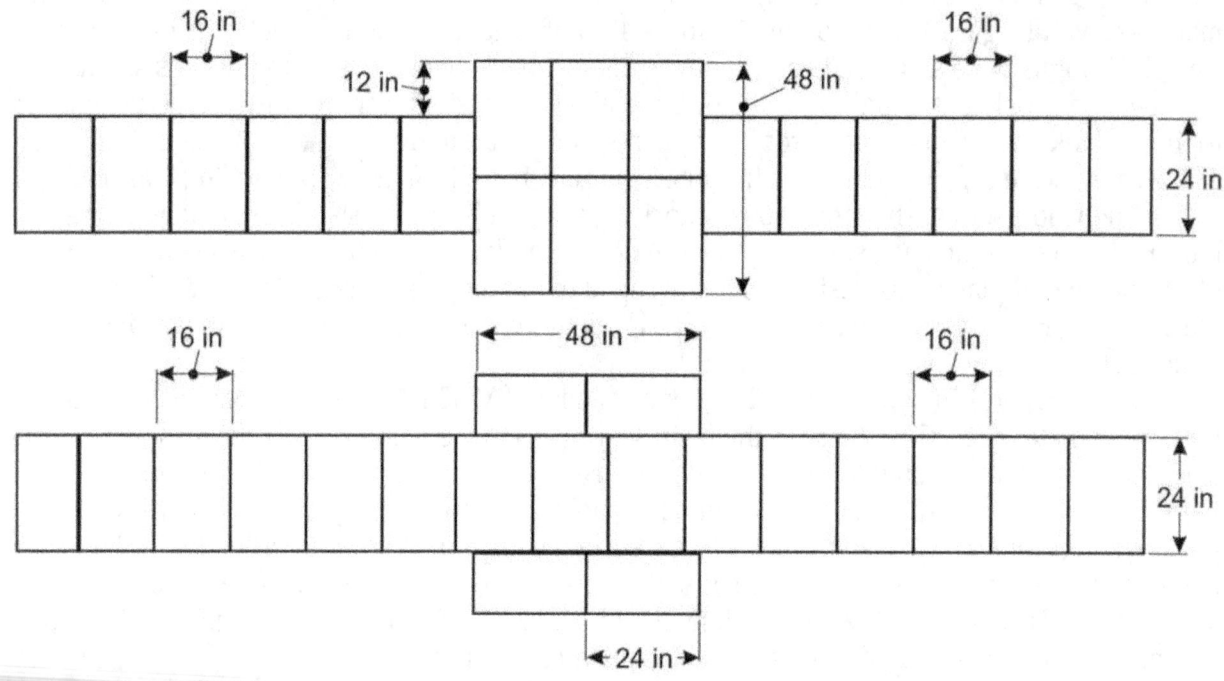

Figure 14.—Schematic of the 24-in-thick, low-density block seal with center pilaster.

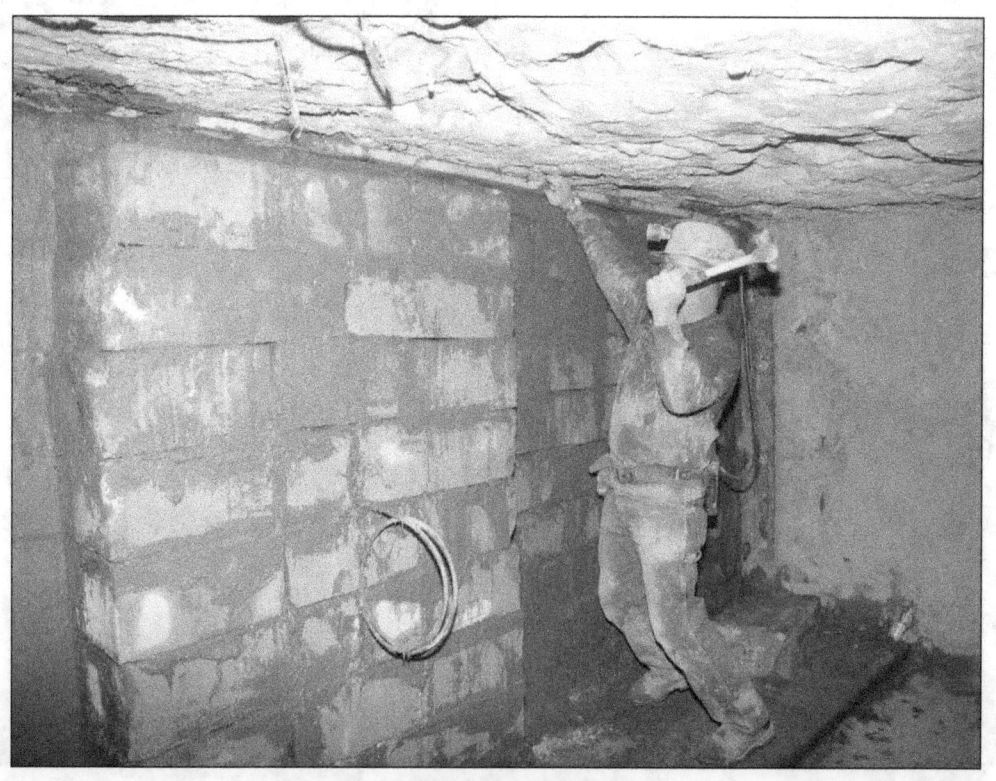

Figure 15.—Installing the wood planking on the top course of block.

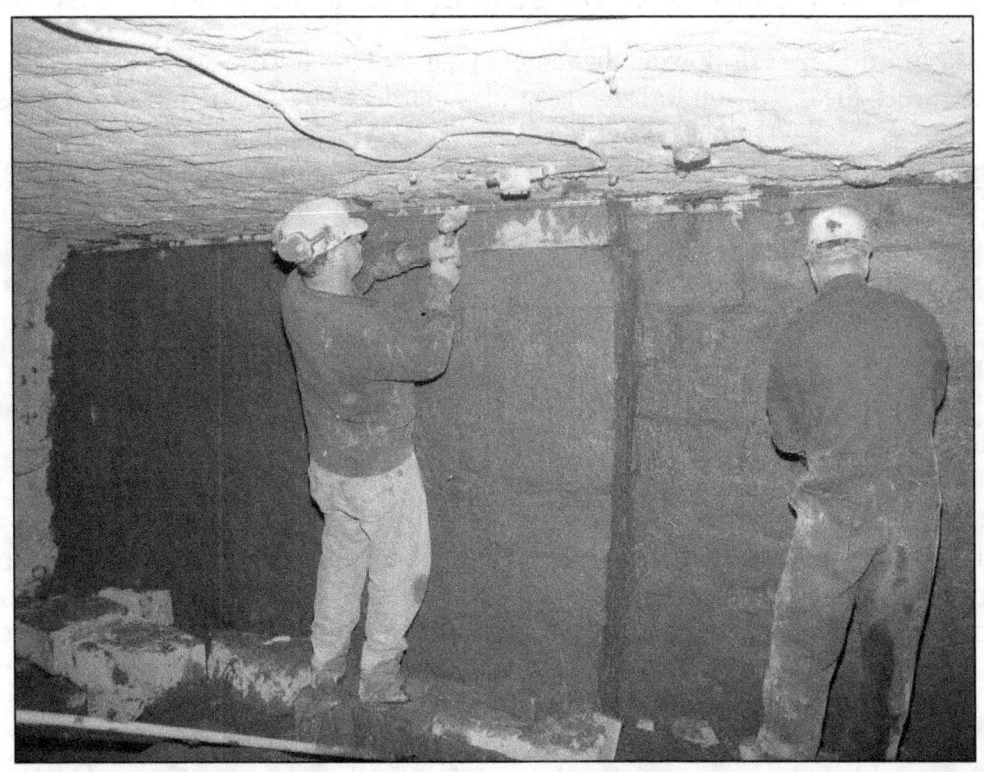

Figure 16.—Wood wedges driven perpendicular between the mine roof and wood planking.

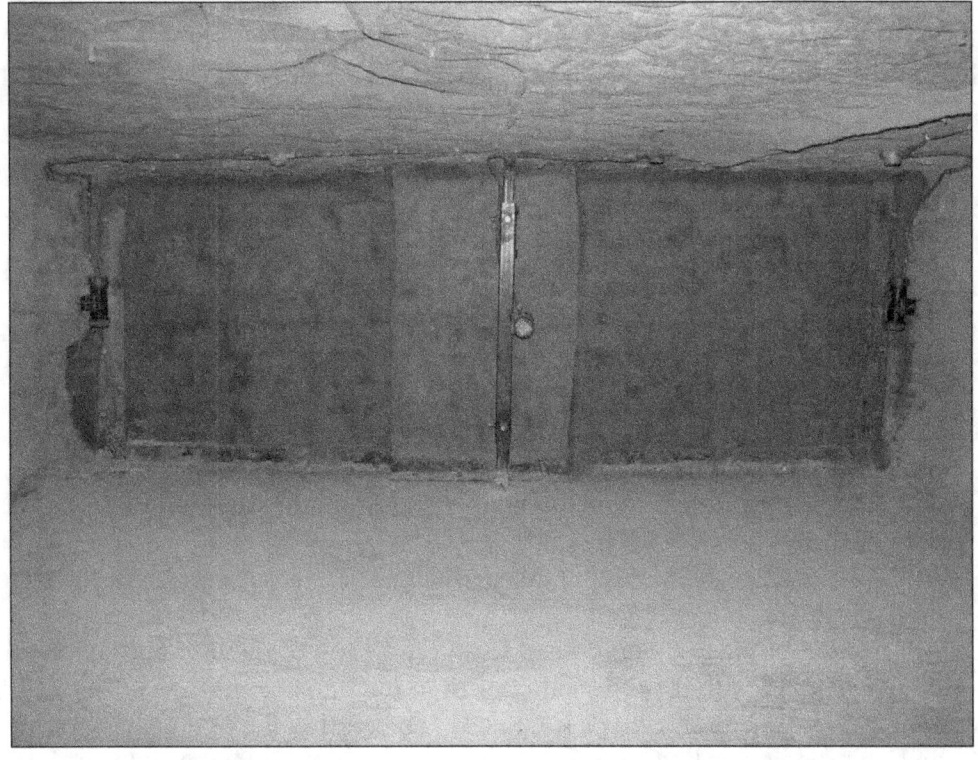

Figure 17.—Completed 24-in-thick, low-density block seal as seen from the C-drift (explosion) side.

CARBON FIBER-REINFORCED POLYMER REINFORCEMENT TECHNIQUE

In early April 2007, following the required curing time for the two constructed alterative 20-psi-rated seals, the CFRP reinforcement retrofit (BlastSeal by Transco Mine Services Co., Chicago, IL) was installed on the outby side of each seal. The outby side refers to the accessible side of the seal in an actual coal mine. For the cementitious pumpable foam seal, the materials necessary to complete the CFRP reinforcement retrofit were installed on the outby side of the C-drift seal. For the low-density block seal in crosscut 3, the materials were installed on the B-drift side. The 50-psi reinforcement upgrades, installed by the manufacturer, were structurally designed to withstand up to an 85-psi reflected pressure generated from a head-on explosion pressure pulse. The CFRP reinforcement retrofit technique was similar for both seals. This reinforcement retrofit was installed by personnel from Sustainable Construction Group, LLC, of Chicago, IL, and Transco Mine Services Co.

Cementitious Pumpable Foam Seal

The materials necessary for the CFRP reinforcement technique were first installed on the 48-in-thick cementitious foam seal located across C-drift at C-320. The exposed sections of brattice, on the outby side of the cementitious seal, were removed. Any cured cementitious foam material that extended beyond the wooden crossboards of the outby framework was chipped away to provide a more uniform roof-to-floor surface.

The 4-in-thick rigid, high-density urethane board (Precision Board PBHT-15, a 4-ft by 8-ft by 4-in thick high-temperature tooling board, 15-lb/ft^3 density, manufactured by Coastal Enterprises, Orange, CA) was installed between the existing 6-in by 4-in wood framework posts of the seal and attached directly to the wooden crossboards with lag screws and 2-in fender washers or 2.5-in metal pin plates. Each section of the rigid urethane board was cut and trimmed to fit between the upright wood posts of the seal framework. The rigid urethane boards were also cut in half, with the bottom half attached first to facilitate construction. The following steps were taken to secure the rigid urethane board to the seal:

(1) Removal of the dust and debris from the mine floor and ribs;
(2) Application of beads of liquid nails to the back of the rigid urethane board;
(3) Spray application of a two-component, 3-lb/ft^3-density polyurethane foam (Touch 'n Seal Foam Kit 120 manufactured by Convenience Products, Fenton, MO) to the concrete mine floor between the wood posts of the seal framework;
(4) Positioning of the bottom section of the rigid urethane board into the high-density foam at the floor;
(5) Securing of the rigid urethane board to the seal by installing lag screws and 2-in fender washers (whose large outside diameter better distributes the forces applied when tightening) or 2.5-in metal pin plates through the rigid urethane board and into the wood crossboards of the seal framework;
(6) Application of beads of liquid nails to the back of the top section of the rigid urethane board;
(7) Application of the two-component foam on the top of the bottom section of rigid urethane board with the top section of rigid urethane board then positioned in place;
(8) Securing of the top section of rigid urethane board to the seal using the lag screws and 2-in fender washers or 2.5-in metal pin plates through the rigid urethane board and into the wood crossboards of the seal framework (Figures 18–19).

Holes were drilled through the rigid urethane board at random locations approximately 12–18 in apart. The two-component foam was injected through the holes, beginning at the bottom, to fill the uneven areas between the urethane board and existing seal surface (Figure 18). The excess two-component foam that expanded out from between the rigid urethane boards, the wood posts, and the roof/floor was then trimmed flush and removed.

After the rigid urethane board was secured to the seal, the first course of 8-in-wide by 6-in-high by 16-in-long solid-concrete block was laid wet using BlocBond. A full bed of BlocBond was applied to the concrete floor, the vertical joints between blocks, and the gaps between the block and ribs. One 50-lb bag of BlocBond was used for this course. (Note that BlocBond was used only on the first course). This first course of block was offset approximately 1 in outby the wood framework posts of the cementitious seal. The concrete blocks were laid with the 8-in block dimension down, and three beads of a one-component polyurethane adhesive (Touch 'n Seal Mine Block Mortar manufactured by Convenience Products, Fenton, MO) were used on all of the joints, with the block joints staggered (Figure 19). After completion of every two to three block courses, the two-component, high-density foam was injected into the approximately 1-in-wide gap between the seal and block wall. As the block wall approached the mine roof, holes were drilled through a few of the solid-concrete blocks to continue the two-component, high-density foam injection in the 1-in-wide gap between the seal and block wall (Figure 20). A total of 15 courses of block were required to complete the wall (206 full blocks plus 21 partial blocks). In several areas, pieces of concrete block and/or the rigid urethane board were cut to size to complete the closure of the course to the mine rib. The two-component foam was then injected into this area to fill all gaps. Wood wedges were used to tighten the block wall to the mine roof. The two-component foam was again used to fill the gaps between the rigid urethane board and concrete block wall.

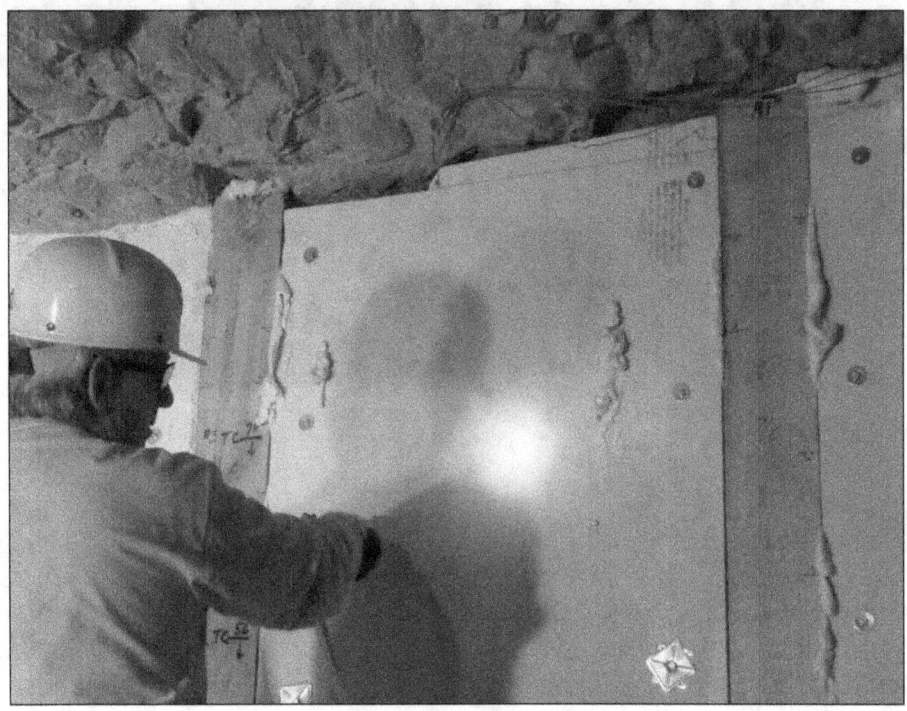

Figure 18.—Injection of the two-component foam behind the rigid urethane board that was secured between the form wall posts with lag screws.

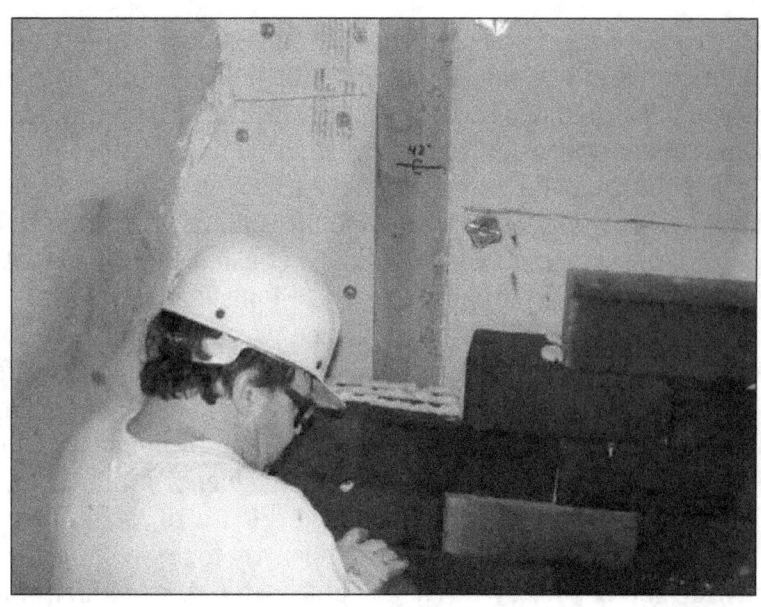

Figure 19.—Construction of the solid-concrete-block wall. A one-component foam adhesive was used on all of the block joints.

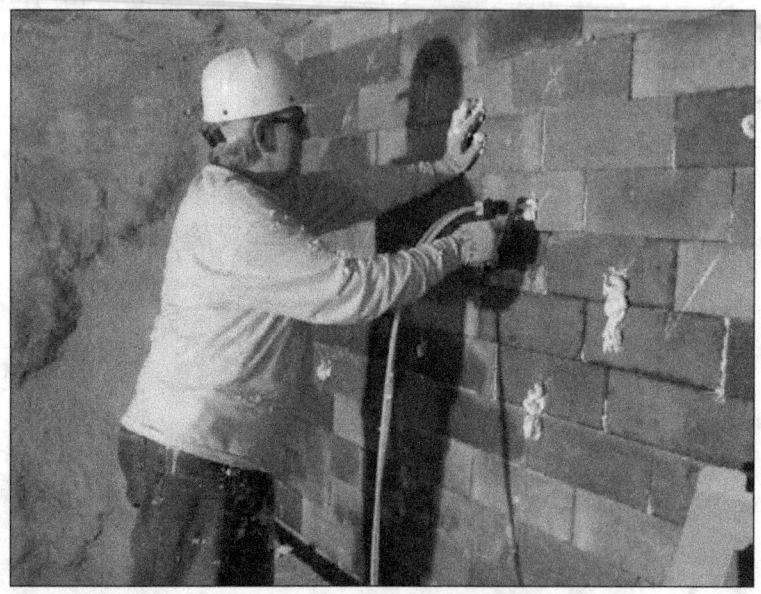

Figure 20.—Injection of the two-component foam through the block to fill the 1-in gap between the seal and concrete block wall.

After completion of the wall, 1 gal of BlastSeal Primer Resin was mixed and painted on the wall using a paint roller. The primer resin was a two-component resin (parts A and B) mixed to a 2A:1B ratio. The primer resin was allowed to cure for 45 min to achieve the proper tackiness. The cure time will vary depending on the temperature and humidity conditions. BlastSeal Tack Resin was then applied on top of the primer resin using a paint roller and smoothed with trowels. The tack resin was a two-component resin (parts A and B) mixed to a 1A:1B ratio. The tack resin was applied only in a sufficiently large area to accommodate the application of the 51-in-wide woven CFRP reinforcement wrap. A total of 4.5 gal of tack resin was used on this seal. Using scissors, the 51-in-wide bidirectional woven CFRP reinforcement BlastSeal base wrap was then cut to size and installed from roof to floor at the center of the block wall. BlastSeal Saturant Resin was then applied to the CFRP base wrap. The saturant resin was a two-component resin (parts A and B) mixed to a 2A:1B ratio. Paint rollers were used to apply the saturant resin coat over the wrap while, at the same time, the wrap was pressed into the tack coat to remove any trapped air bubbles behind the wrap. Additional panels of base wrap were installed in a similar manner with a 6-in overlap to the previous panel wrap until the entire face of the block wall was covered (Figure 21). Figure 22 shows the woven CFRP base wrap being cut to match the contour of the mine rib and roof. A total of six panels of the bidirectional CFRP base wrap were required to cover the concrete block wall. A total of 3.5 gal of the saturant resin was used to coat the base wrap. A second unidirectional woven CFRP BlastSeal finish wrap was then applied over the base wrap so that the high-strength carbon fibers were installed in the vertical direction. The finish wrap was coated with the saturant resin. Each panel of the finish wrap was centered roof to floor over the panel joints of the base wrap. A total of 4 gal of the saturant resin was used to coat the unidirectional finish wrap. The wraps did not overlap on the roof, ribs, or floor.

Two 9-ft-long sections of 6-in by 6-in by ½-in thick steel angle (ASTM A–36) were then anchored on 12-in centers across the roof and similarly across the floor using 1-in-diam by 12-in long Hilti Kwik Bolt III anchor bolts (for coal mine applications, different bolts would be required to provide equivalent anchorage strength). All gaps between the steel angle and roof and the steel angle and seal were filled with the high-strength mortar (BlocBond). Figure 23 shows the C–320 pumpable cementitious foam seal with the completed CFRP reinforcement retrofit. The average mine temperature was ~59 °F with an average relative humidity of ~83% during the time required to install the CFRP reinforcement retrofit at the C–320 seal.

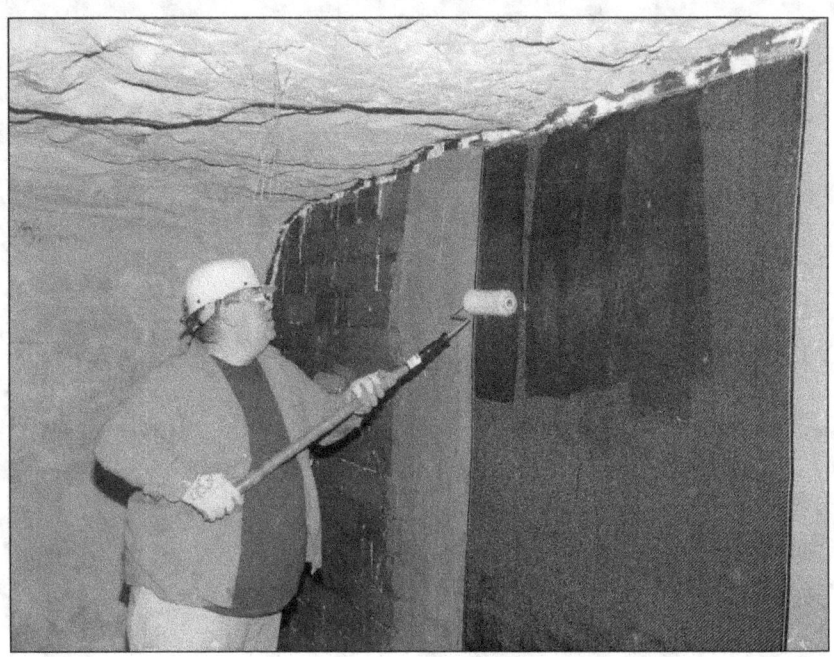

Figure 21.—Applying the resin saturant coat over the CFRP base wrap.
The light gray undercoating on the concrete block is the resin tack.

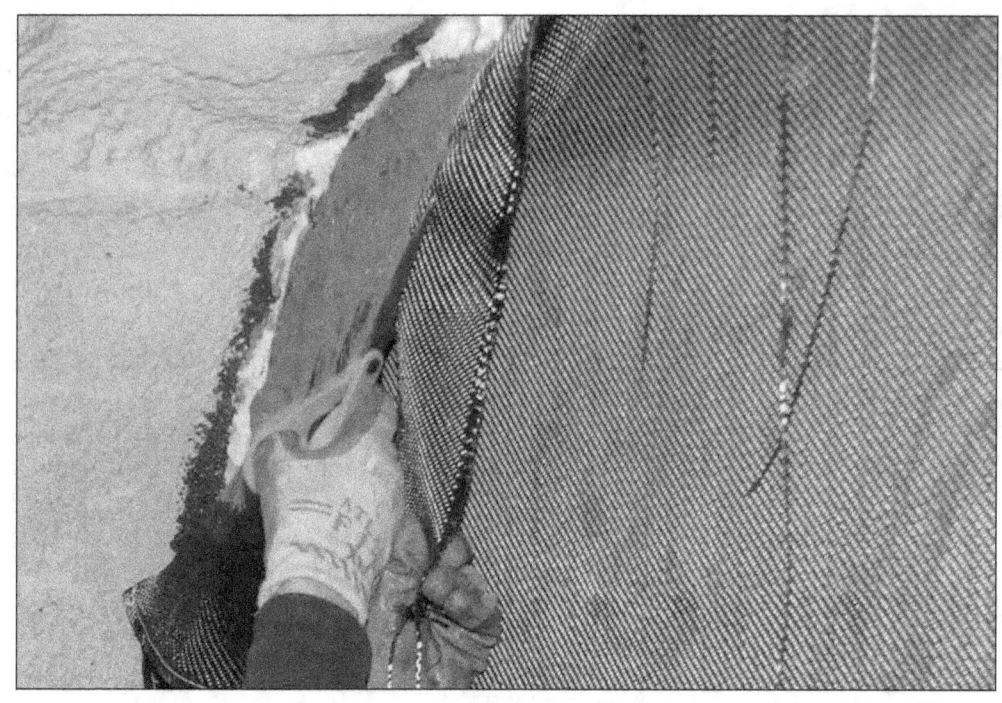

Figure 22.—Cutting the woven CFRP base wrap to match the contour of the mine rib and roof.

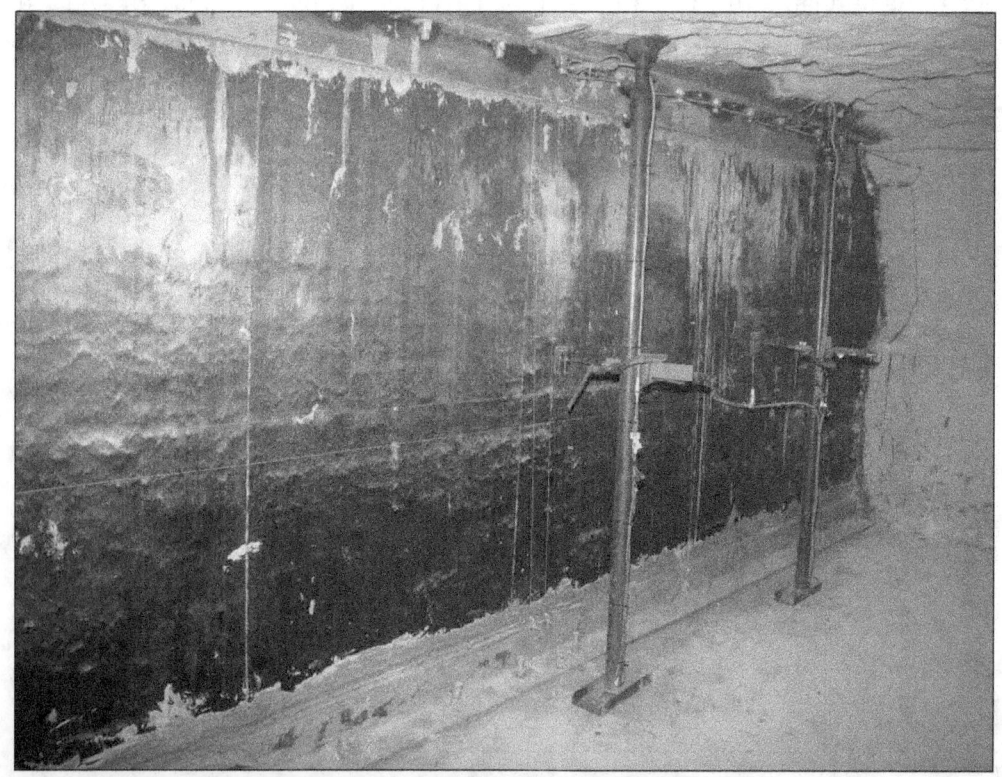

Figure 23.—Completed CFRP reinforcement retrofit to the C–320 pumpable cementitious foam seal, and the LVDT displacement sensors mounted to posts and attached to seal.

Low-Density Block Seal

The CFRP reinforcement retrofit for the 24-in-thick, low-density block seal with a center pilaster (48 in by 48 in) located in crosscut 3 was constructed in a manner similar to that of the cementitious pumpable seal. The 4-in-thick, rigid, high-density urethane board was installed on each side of the seal's center pilaster and attached directly to the seal. The following steps were taken to secure the rigid urethane board to the seal:

(1) Removal of the dust and debris from the mine floor and ribs;
(2) Cutting and positioning of the rigid urethane board for as tight a fit as possible to the roof and floor (Figure 24);
(3) Securing of the rigid urethane board to the seal by positioning 2-in by 4-in boards onto the rigid urethane board and wedging it in place against a roof jack.

Holes were then drilled through the rigid urethane board for injection of the two-component foam (Touch 'n Seal Foam Kit 120). The foam was used to fill, until refusal, the voids between the seal and the back of the rigid urethane boards (Figure 25). The two-component foam expanded from between the rigid urethane boards, sides, and the roof/floor, which held the board in place when the 2×4 bracing was removed. The excess foam was then trimmed flush with adjoining surfaces.

After the rigid urethane board was secured to the seal with the two-component, high-density foam, the concrete block walls on each side of the center pilaster were constructed in the same manner as for the seal across C-drift. A total of 13 full courses of block were required to complete the wall (136 full blocks plus 26 partial blocks) on either side of the pilaster. For the top course of each block wall, half (4-in by 8-in by 16-in solid) and cap (2-in by 8-in by 16-in solid) blocks were used to provide a tighter fit to the mine roof. Wood wedges were used to tighten the block wall to the mine roof. Wedges were temporarily used at the ribs to tighten each block course, but were later removed after the one-component foam adhesive (Touch 'n Seal Mine Block Mortar) between the blocks cured (Figure 26). The two-component foam was then injected to fill all gaps between the block and at the perimeter.

The woven CFRP base and finish wraps were installed in a similar manner as the C–320 cementitious pumpable seal. After completion of the wall sections, 1.5 gal of primer resin was mixed and painted on the pilaster and two concrete block walls using a paint roller (Figure 27). The tack resin was then applied on top of the primer resin using a paint roller and smoothed with trowels. A total of 4.5 gal of tack resin was used on this seal. The 51-in-wide bidirectional woven CFRP base wrap was then cut to size and installed from roof to floor starting at the center of the pilaster. The saturant resin was then applied to the CFRP base wrap. Additional panels of base wrap were installed in a similar manner with a 6-in overlap to the previous panel wrap until the entire face of the pilaster and two concrete block walls were covered. A total of five panels of the base wrap were required to cover the pilaster and concrete block walls. A total of 3.5 gal of the saturant resin was used to coat the base wrap. A second unidirectional woven CFRP finish wrap was then applied over the base wrap so that the high-strength carbon fibers were also installed in the vertical direction. The finish wrap was coated with the saturant resin. Each panel of the finish wrap was centered roof to floor over the panel joints of the base wrap. A total of 4 gal of the saturant resin was used to coat the finish wrap. The wraps did not overlap on the roof, ribs, or floor. Two 9-ft-long sections of 6-in by 6-in by ½-in thick steel angle (ASTM A–36) were then anchored on 12-in centers across the roof and similarly across the floor (shorter angle pieces were used on the floor since the 4-ft-wide pilaster already had bolted steel angle to simulate floor hitching) using 1-in-diam by 12-in-long Kwik Bolt III anchor bolts. All gaps between the steel angle and roof and the steel angle and seal were filled with the high-strength mortar (BlocBond). Figure 28 shows the completed CFRP reinforcement retrofit application to the crosscut 3 seal. The average mine temperature was ~60 °F with an average relative humidity of ~71% during the retrofit installation on the low-density block seal in crosscut 3.

Approximately 16 hr were required to complete the retrofit upgrade to the pumpable cementitious foam seal and about 12 hr for the low-density block seal. However, it is anticipated that as personnel become more familiar with the construction techniques, the total upgrade installation time will require 8–10 hr per seal.

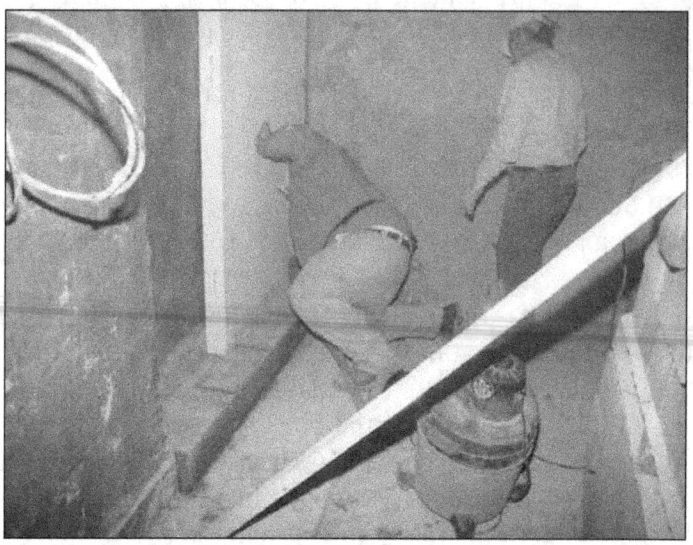

Figure 24.—Positioning the rigid urethane board between the first course of concrete block and the seal.

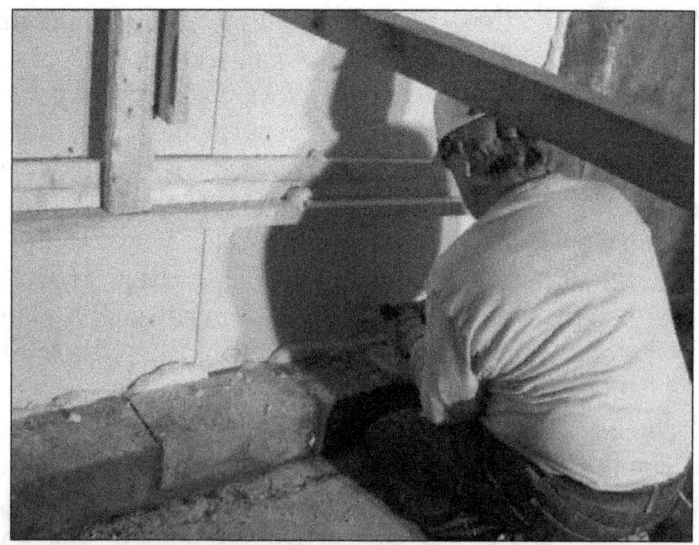

Figure 25.—Injection of the two-component polyurethane foam at the perimeter and behind the rigid urethane board.

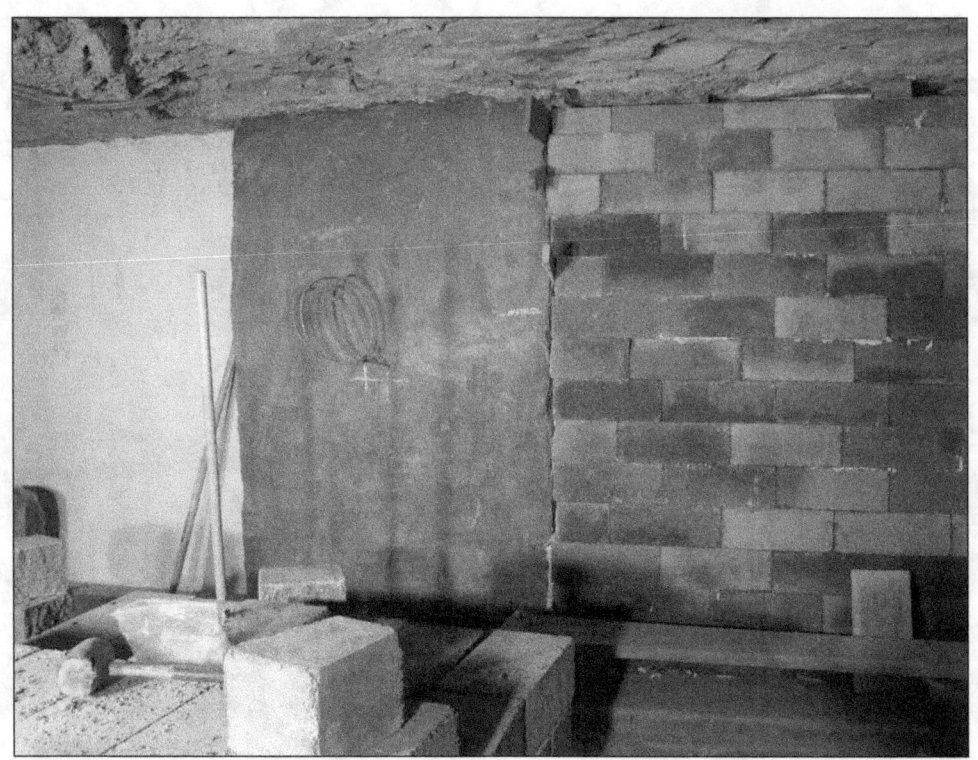

Figure 26.—Completed block wall to the right of the pilaster and the installed rigid urethane board to the left.

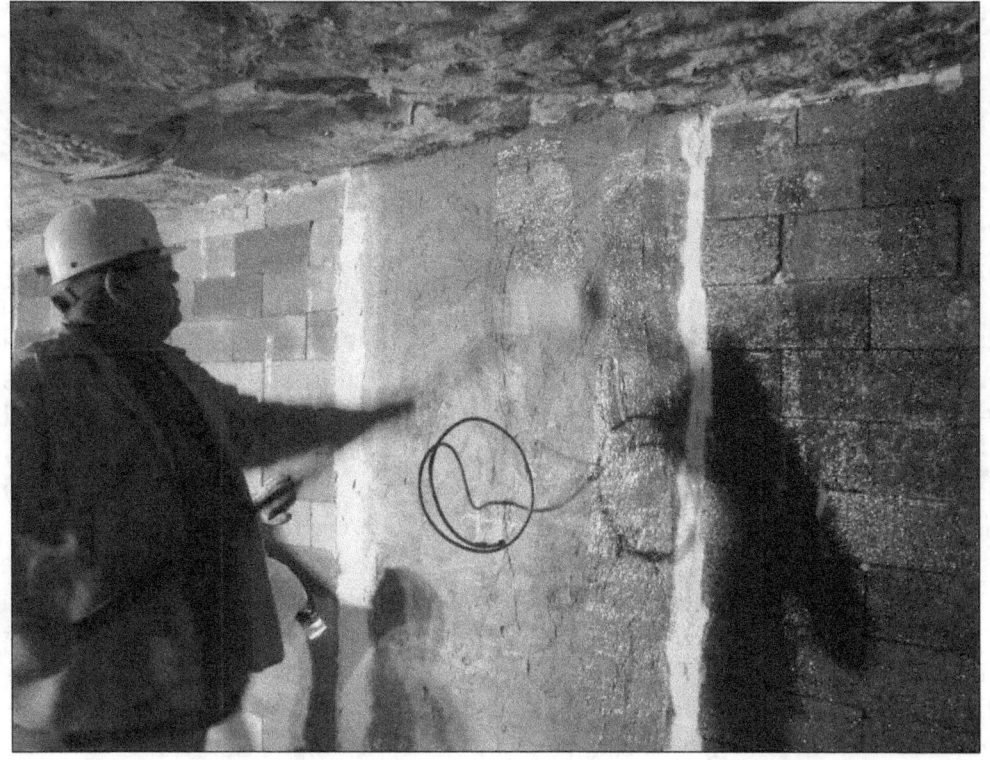

Figure 27.—Applying the primer resin with a paint roller to the concrete block and pilaster.

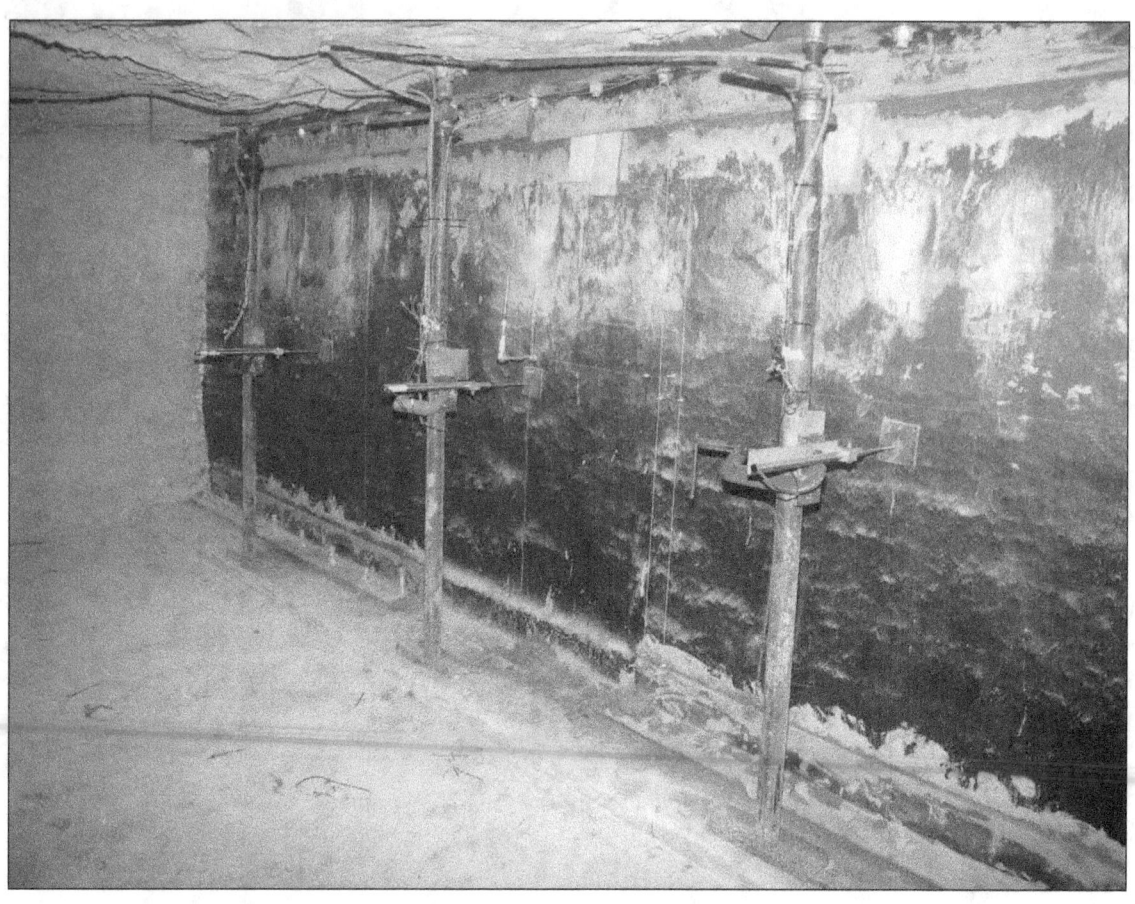

Figure 28.—Completed CFRP reinforcement retrofit to the crosscut 3 low-density block seal.

EXPLOSION TEST RESULTS

Preexplosion air leakage measurements on the seals showed no detectable leakages at either seal at pressure differentials up to 4.3 in H_2O (Table 1). Figure 29 is a schematic of the test setup for the CFRP reinforcement retrofit mine seal evaluations in the LLEM. The difference between the test setup shown in Figure 29 and that shown in Figure 2 is that a seal is now installed across C-drift between crosscuts 3 and 4, thereby confining the explosion pressures. For the first explosion test (LLEM test 508), a gas ignition zone was confined by a plastic diaphragm across C-drift at 47 ft from the face (Figures 2 and 29). About 661 ft^3 of natural gas was injected into the ignition zone to produce a mixture of approximately 10% methane-in-air. The flammable gas was ignited using the triple-point ignition source. The pressure pulse propagated out C-drift past the seals in crosscuts 1, 2, and 3. This test method is essentially the same as that used during the LLEM seal tests during the 1990s and early 2000s [Stephan 1990a,b; Greninger et al. 1991; Weiss et al. 1993a,b,c; 1996; 1997; 1999; 2002]. However in this test, the explosion was confined by the seal located across C-drift at 320 ft, and the pressures were built up higher than in the past tests. The seals in the crosscuts experienced the side-on sweeping explosion pressure pulse, and the seal in C-drift experienced the head-on explosion pressure pulse.

Table 1.—Air leakage measurements before the first explosion test (LLEM test 508)

Location	Air leakage rates, cfm, at pressure differential of—			
	0.8 in H$_2$O	1.4 in H$_2$O	2.3 in H$_2$O	4.3 in H$_2$O
Retrofitted seal in crosscut 3..................	0	0	0	0
Retrofitted seal across C-drift (C–320) ...	0	0	0	0

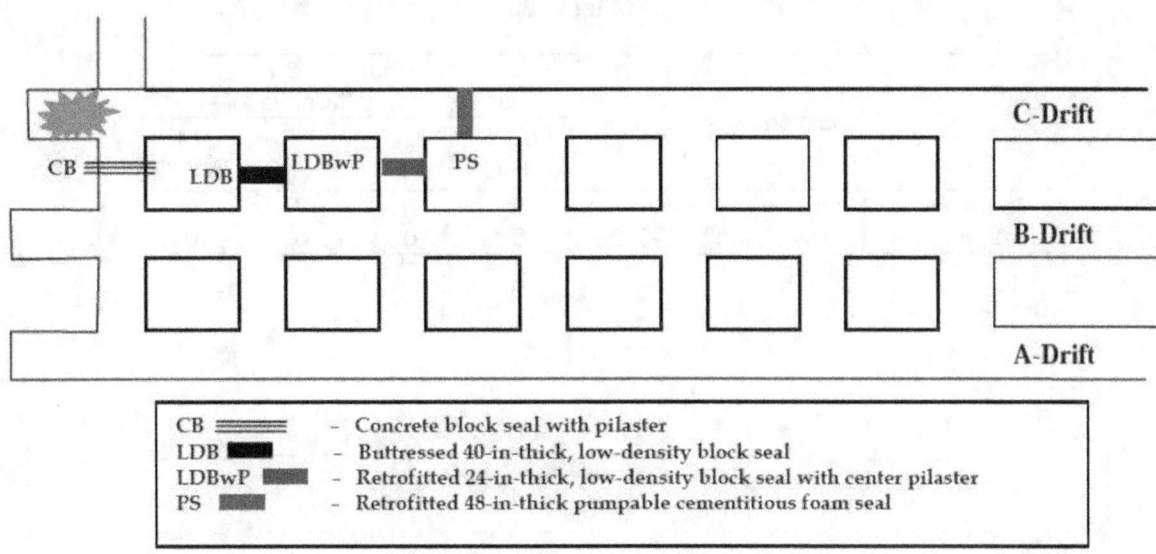

Figure 29.—Test setup for the mine seal retrofit evaluations in the LLEM.

The first explosion test generated an initial outgoing side-on (or sweeping) explosion pressure of approximately 28 psi (at ~0.58 sec) at the retrofitted low-density block seal in crosscut 3 (Figure 30). The head-on explosion at the retrofitted cementitious pumpable foam seal at C–320 generated a reflected peak explosion pressure of 61 psi (Figure 31). As can be seen in Figure 30, a subsequent 36-psi peak side-on explosion pressure at ~0.68 sec was generated at the retrofitted low-density block seal in crosscut 3 due to the reflected pressure pulse from the C–320 seal. These explosion pressure data are for horizontally mounted transducers at the middle front of the seals, and the data are averaged over 10 ms. Both seals with the CFRP reinforcement retrofit survived the explosion. Additional details of the pressure data generated during test 1 (LLEM test 508) are presented in Table A–1 in the Appendix.

Behind each seal was an LVDT mounted to the posts, as shown in Figure 4. The LVDT measures the movement of the seal during the explosion. The C–320 seal exhibited a permanent displacement of approximately ½ in (represented by curves at the top of Figure 31). The crosscut 3 seal exhibited a permanent displacement of approximately 0.04 in (represented by curves at the top of Figure 30).

Postexplosion air leakage measurements were then collected on each seal. The crosscut 3 seal had no detectable leakage. The C–320 seal exhibited only negligible leakage when subjected to pressure differentials up to 4.1 in H_2O (Table 2).

Table 2.—Air leakage measurements after the first explosion test
(LLEM test 508)

Location	Air leakage rates, cfm, at pressure differential of—			
	0.8 in H_2O	1.4 in H_2O	2.2 in H_2O	4.1 in H_2O
Retrofitted seal in crosscut 3....................	0	0	0	0
Retrofitted seal across C-drift (C–320) ...	0	0	0	0

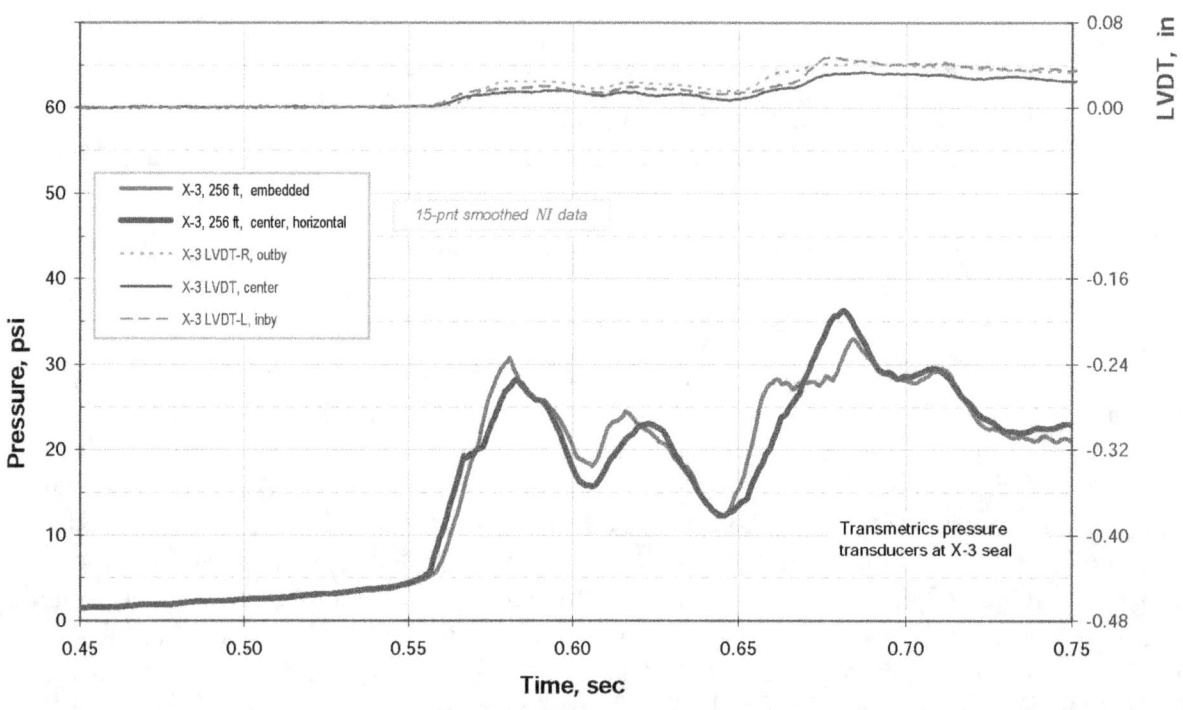

Figure 30.—Pressures and LVDT displacements at the crosscut 3 seal during test 1 (LLEM test 508).

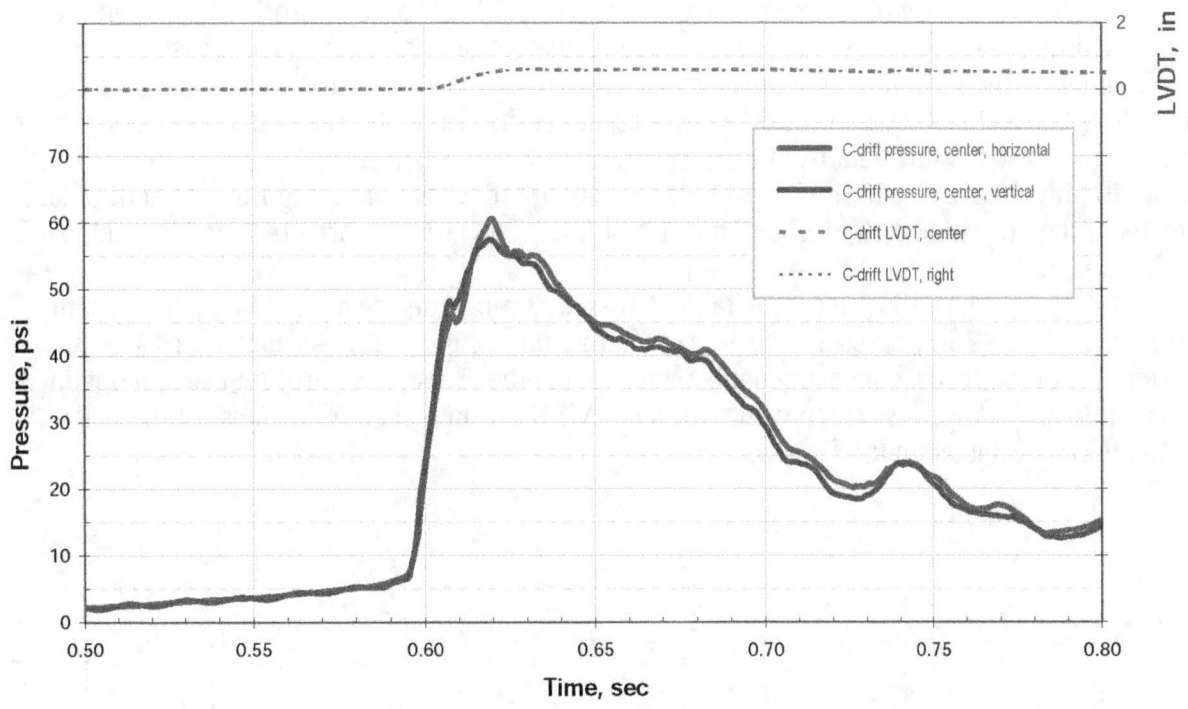

Figure 31.—Pressures and LVDT displacements at the C–320 seal during test 1 (LLEM test 508).

A second explosion test (LLEM test 509) was then conducted to generate a higher explosion pressure at the retrofitted low-density block seal in crosscut 3. A longer 71-ft gas ignition zone was used at the face of C-drift. In this test, the plastic diaphragm used to confine the gas mixture was located just outby crosscut 1. The 71-ft ignition zone was filled with 1,265 ft^3 of natural gas to give a mixture of ~10% methane-in-air. Although this zone was only ~50% longer than the ignition zone for the first test (LLEM test 508), the flammable gas volume was ~90% greater. This was due to the additional volume in crosscut 1 between the seal and the bulkhead door leading to E-drift, as shown in Figures 2 and 29. Additionally, 8 lb of pulverized coal dust was loaded on shelves suspended from the mine roof at four locations outby the end of the ignition zone. These shelves were located at 77, 87, 97, and 107 ft from the closed end. The flammable methane-air zone was ignited using the triple-point ignition source at the face of C-drift, and the explosion pressure pulse propagated out C-drift past the seals in crosscuts 1 through 3 to the seal in C-drift. The seals in the crosscuts experienced the side-on explosion pressures, and the seal in C-drift experienced the head-on explosion pressure. Because the flammable gas zone was much larger and 32 lb of pulverized coal dust was used, the resulting explosion pressures were much higher than those in the first test. To achieve the desired explosion pressure at the retrofitted low-density block seal in crosscut 3 during the second test, the explosion pressures at the retrofitted C–320 seal would be well in excess of the 85-psi design strength of the CFRP reinforcement retrofit as installed on the pumpable cementitious foam seal.

The total explosion pressure at the C–320 seal was ~132 psi (reflected pressure resulting from the head-on explosion) as recorded at the center of the seal, and the seal was destroyed as expected (Figure 32). The low-density block seal with the CFRP reinforcement retrofit in crosscut 3 survived the explosion. The initial outgoing pressure wave generated a side-on sweeping pressure pulse of approximately 50 psi (at ~0.49 sec) at the retrofitted low-density block seal in crosscut 3 (Figure 33). The cables to the pressure transducers at crosscut 3 were severed before the peak reflected pressure traveling back inby from the C–320 seal could be recorded. The estimated side-on explosion pressure at the crosscut 3 retrofitted seal was greater than 60 psi, based on the data from the pressure transducer in a nearby DG station located on the mine rib inby the seal location (C–234 ft, wall pressure trace shown in Figure 33). Additional details of the pressure data generated during test 2 (LLEM test 509) are presented in Table A–2 in the Appendix.

Based on the LVDT sensor data, the crosscut 3 retrofitted seal exhibited a permanent displacement of ~2 in (represented by curves at the top of Figure 33). As shown in Table 3, postexplosion air leakage measurements revealed that the crosscut 3 retrofitted seal maintained acceptable air leakage resistance well within the MSHA-established guidelines for the seal evaluations conducted in the LLEM.

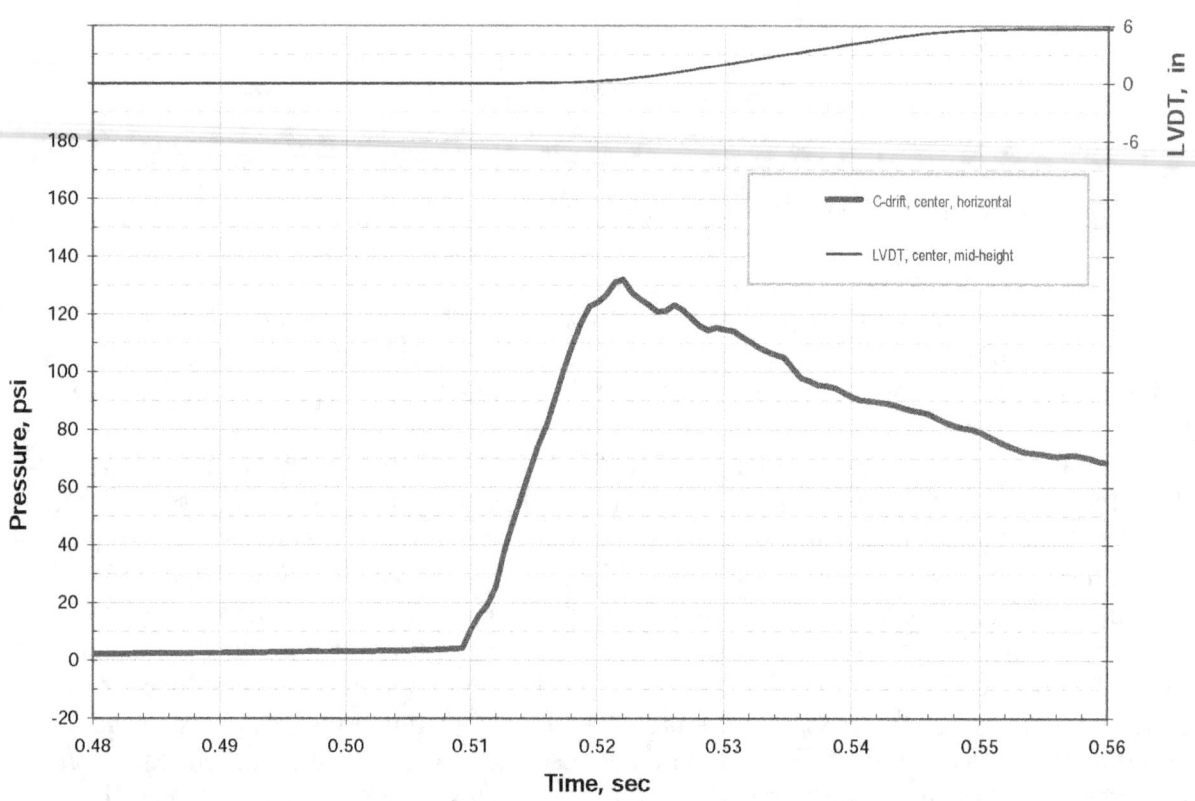

Figure 32.—Pressures and LVDT displacements at the C–320 seal during test 2 (LLEM test 509).

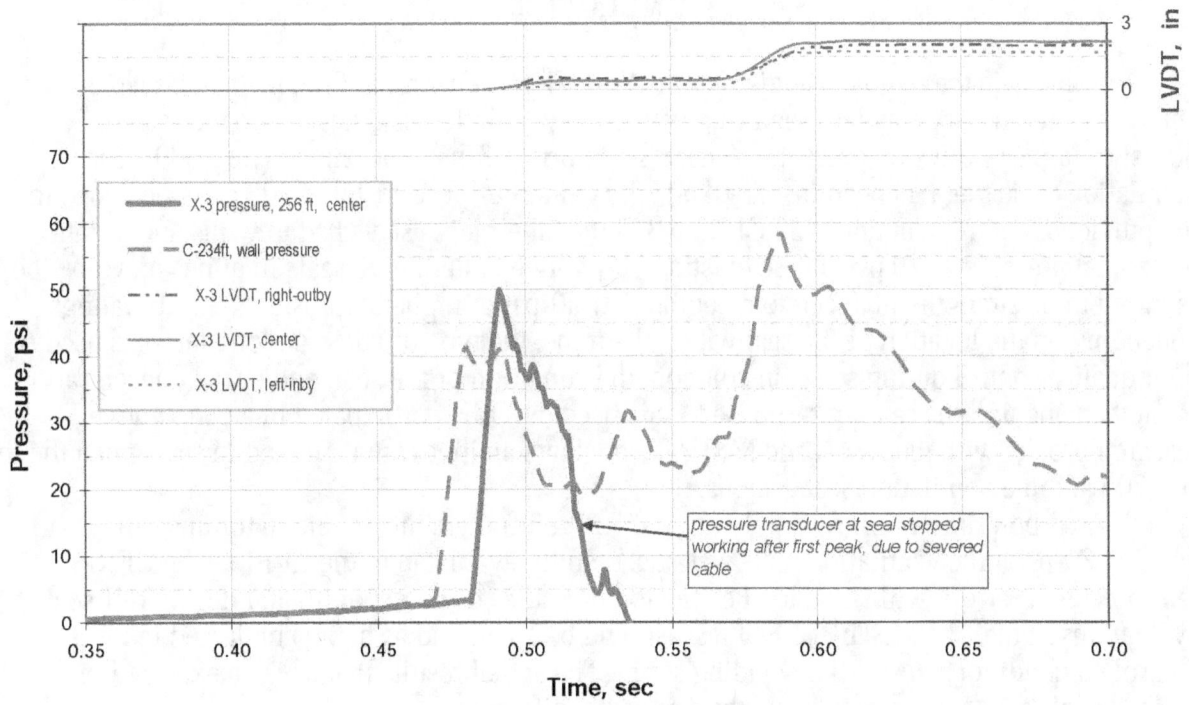

Figure 33.—Pressures and LVDT displacements at the crosscut 3 seal during test 2 (LLEM test 509).

Table 3.—Air leakage measurements after the second explosion test (LLEM test 509)

Location	Air leakage rates, cfm, at pressure differential of—			
	0.55 in H₂O	1.0 in H₂O	1.8 in H₂O	3.7 in H₂O
Buttressed seal in crosscut 2....................	19	28	37	56
Retrofitted seal in crosscut 3	24	35	47	70
Retrofitted seal across C-drift (C–320)	Seal destroyed.			

CONCLUSIONS

Following the Sago Mine disaster in West Virginia in early 2006, MSHA issued an emergency temporary standard requiring new mine ventilation seal designs to withstand 50-psi or higher explosion pressures. The vast majority of the approximately 14,000 mine ventilation seals that had been installed in U.S. coal mines prior to July 2006 were designed to the previous requirement under 30 CFR 75.335 that alternative seals had to withstand a static horizontal pressure of 20 psi. These existing 20-psi-rated alternative seals in mines may now be required to be strength-enhanced to meet the new 50-psi or higher explosion pressure ratings depending on the location of the seal within the mine, the type of construction materials used, poor quality control during seal construction, the condition of the seal, and/or the concentration of methane behind the seal. In response to this need, NIOSH participated in a cooperative research project with the NMA and MSHA to evaluate an innovative method to strengthen the in situ 20-psi mine ventilation seal designs.

A carbon fiber-reinforced polymer (CFRP) reinforcement technique for upgrading existing 20-psi mine ventilation seals was successfully evaluated in the LLEM. The CFRP reinforcement retrofit withstood total explosion pressures of 60 psi or greater during full-scale evaluations in the LLEM. The LLEM tests should be construed as being conducted in ideal, controlled conditions in solid, unyielding strata. The actual results that may be expected in various coal mine environments may be somewhat different.

Several variations of the CFRP reinforcement technique for upgrading existing 20-psi-rated seals have been recently deemed suitable by MSHA for use in underground coal mines, including two 120-psi upgrade designs. Several other upgrade designs are currently in the technical review process and under development by the manufacturer.

NIOSH will continue to evaluate new, innovative retrofit techniques for addressing the strength adequacy issues associated with existing seals in coal mines. Strengthening existing 20-psi mine ventilation seals to withstand 50-psi or greater explosion pressures will result in a significant reduction in the failure rates of these seals, thereby enhancing the safety of miners in the active areas of underground coal mines.

ACKNOWLEDGMENTS

The authors thank Adam K. P. Brown, Project Manager and Safety Director, Transco Mine Services Co., for taking the initiative, in the wake of the Sago and Darby Mine No. 1 disasters in 2006, to develop a partnership for adapting the CFRP reinforcement techniques used in other industries to the underground coal mining industry. Together, the partnership members designed a strength-enhancing upgrade for existing mine ventilation seals that better withstands the explosion overpressures resulting from ignitions within the sealed area, thereby improving the safety of underground coal miners. We thank the following personnel associated with this partnership for their roles in the design of the CFRP reinforcement technique, materials, and/or installations within the LLEM: Edward J. Wolbert, President/CEO, and J. Michael Sollie of Transco Products, Inc.; George A. Mathes, P.E., CEO, First Defense, LLC, Phoenix, AZ; Ravi Kanitkar, Senior Structural Engineer, P.E., Associate, Crosby Group, Redwood City, CA; Jim Butler, President, HJ3 Composite Technologies, Tucson, AZ; John O'Leary, Vice President Special Projects, Coatings Unlimited, Inc., St. Louis, MO; and Timothy R. Ervin, Mark Luhn, Michael P. Boner, and Joshua W. G. Hamm of Sustainable Construction Group, LLC, St. Louis, MO.

The authors also thank the NMA and its members Bruce Watzman, Vice President, Safety and Health, Washington, DC; Philip Molesky of CONSOL Energy, Inc., Scenery Hill, PA; John Gallick of Foundation Coal Co., Waynesburg, PA; and Doug Conaway of Arch Coal, Inc., St. Louis, MO, for their support and guidance and for providing funding for the materials required to install the seal retrofits. In addition, we thank the following MSHA personnel for their technical guidance and support during this program: Richard A. Allwes, Darren J. Blank, Michael C. Superfesky, and Carol L. Tasillo, Civil Engineers; Terence M. Taylor, Senior Civil Engineer; and Kelvin K. Wu, Ph.D., Chief (now retired), Mine Waste and Geotechnical Engineering Division, Technical Support, Pittsburgh, PA.

The authors acknowledge the following mechanical technicians with Ki Corp. (a NIOSH contractor) for the construction of the low-density block seal, assistance in the underground materials handling, and the extensive cleanup operations: James D. Addis, Timothy W. Glad, James R. Rabon, and Bernard T. Lambie.

In addition, the authors acknowledge the following NIOSH–PRL personnel without whose contributions this program could not have been accomplished: Kenneth L. Cashdollar, Principal Research Scientist, for data analyses and photography; Kenneth W. Jackson, Electronics Technician, for sensor calibrations and installations and for his participation in the testing, data collection, and analyses; Cynthia A. Hollerich, Physical Science Technician, for written and photographic documentation of the seal constructions; Richard A. Thomas, Electronics Technician, and John Soles, Physical Science Technician, for installing thermocouples and documenting the temperature data during the cure period for the pumpable cementitious foam seal; and William A. Slivensky, Frank A. Karnack, and Donald D. Sellers, Physical Science Technicians, for their extensive participation in the installation of the sensors and mounting equipment, explosion and air leakage testing, and construction monitoring.

All photographs in this report were taken by Cynthia A. Hollerich, Kenneth L. Cashdollar, and Eric S. Weiss of NIOSH–PRL.

REFERENCES

72 Fed. Reg. 28795 [2007]. Mine Safety and Health Administration, 30 CFR part 75: sealing of abandoned areas; emergency temporary standard.

CFR. Code of federal regulations. Washington DC: U.S. Government Printing Office, Office of the Federal Register.

Gates RA, Phillips RL, Urosek JE, Stephan CR, Stoltz RT, Swentosky DJ, Harris GW, O'Donnell JR Jr., Dresch RA [2007]. Report of investigation, fatal underground coal mine explosion, January 2, 2006. Sago mine, Wolf Run Mining Company, Tallmansville, Upshur County, West Virginia, ID No. 46–08791. Arlington, VA: U.S. Department of Labor, Mine Safety and Health Administration.

Greninger NB, Weiss ES, Luzik SJ, Stephan CR [1991]. Evaluation of solid-block and cementitious foam Seals. Pittsburgh, PA: U.S. Department of the Interior, Bureau of Mines, RI 9382. NTIS No. PB 92–152115.

Mattes RH, Bacho A, Wade LV [1983]. Lake Lynn Laboratory: construction, physical description, and capability. Pittsburgh, PA: U.S. Department of the Interior, Bureau of Mines, IC 8911. NTIS No. PB 83–197103.

Nagy J [1981]. The explosion hazard in mining. Pittsburgh, PA: U.S. Department of Labor, Mine Safety and Health Administration, IR 1119.

Sapko MJ, Weiss ES, Watson RW [1987]. Size scaling of gas explosions: Bruceton experimental mine versus the Lake Lynn mine. Pittsburgh, PA: U.S. Department of Interior, Bureau of Mines, RI 9136. NTIS No. PB 88–230248.

Stephan CR [1990a]. Construction of seals in underground coal mines. Pittsburgh, PA: U.S. Department of Labor, Mine Safety and Health Administration, Industrial Safety Division (ISD) report No. 06–213–90, August 1, 1990.

Stephan CR [1990b]. Omega 384 block as a seal construction material. Pittsburgh, PA: U.S. Department of Labor, Mine Safety and Health Administration, Industrial Safety Division (ISD) report No. 10–318–90, November 14, 1990.

Triebsch G, Sapko MJ [1990]. Lake Lynn Laboratory: a state-of-the-art mining research laboratory. In: Proceedings of the International Symposium on Unique Underground Structures. Vol. 2. Golden, CO: Colorado School of Mines, pp. 75–1 to 75–21.

Weiss ES, Greninger NB, Perry JW, Stephan CR [1993a]. Strength and leakage evaluations for coal mine seals. In: Proceedings of the 25th International Conference of Safety in Mines Research Institutes (Pretoria, South Africa, September 13–17, 1993), Conference Papers for Day One, pp. 149-161.

Weiss ES, Greninger NB, Slivensky WA, Stephan CR [1993b]. Evaluation of alternative seal designs for coal mines. In: Proceedings of the Sixth U.S. Mine Ventilation Symposium (Salt Lake City, UT, June 21–23, 1993). Chapter 97. Littleton, CO: Society for Mining, Metallurgy, and Exploration, Inc., pp. 635–640.

Weiss ES, Greninger NB, Stephan CR, Lipscomb JR [1993c]. Strength characteristics and air-leakage determinations for alternative mine seal designs. Pittsburgh, PA: U.S. Department of the Interior, Bureau of Mines, RI 9477. NTIS No. PB94111275.

Weiss ES, Slivensky WA, Schultz MJ, Stephan CR, Jackson KW [1996]. Evaluation of polymer construction material and water trap designs for underground coal mine seals. Pittsburgh, PA: U.S. Department of Energy, RI 9634. NTIS No. PB96–123392.

Weiss ES, Slivensky WA, Schultz MJ, Stephan CR [1997]. Evaluation of water trap designs and alternative mine seal construction materials. In: Dhar BB, Bhowmick BC, eds. Proceedings of the 27th International Conference of Safety in Mines Research Institutes (New Delhi, India, February 20–22, 1997). Vol. II. New Delhi, India: Oxford & IBH Publishing Co. Pvt. Ltd., pp. 973–981.

Weiss ES, Cashdollar KL, Mutton IVS, Kohli DR, Slivensky WA [1999]. Evaluation of reinforced cementitious seals. Pittsburgh, PA: U.S. Department of Health and Human Services, Public Health Service, Centers for Disease Control and Prevention, National Institute for Occupational Safety and Health, DHHS (NIOSH) Publication No. 99–136, RI 9647.

Weiss ES, Cashdollar KL, Sapko MJ [2002]. Evaluation of explosion-resistant seals, stoppings, and overcast for ventilation control in underground coal mining. Pittsburgh, PA: U.S. Department of Health and Human Services, Public Health Service, Centers for Disease Control and Prevention, National Institute for Occupational Safety and Health, DHHS (NIOSH) Publication No. 2003–104, RI 9659.

Zipf RK Jr., Sapko MJ, Brune JF [2007]. Explosion pressure design criteria for new seals in U.S. coal mines. Pittsburgh, PA: U.S. Department of Health and Human Services, Public Health Service, Centers for Disease Control and Prevention, National Institute for Occupational Safety and Health, DHHS (NIOSH) Publication No. 2007–144, IC 9500.

APPENDIX.—SUMMARY TABLES OF PRESSURE DATA FOR LLEM EXPLOSION TESTS

Table A–1.—Maximum wall and seal pressures during test 1 (LLEM test 508)

WALL PRESSURES				
B-drift			C-drift	
Distance	Pressure		Distance	Pressure
ft	psi		ft	psi
10	0.03		13	27.6
108	0.04		84	25.4
158	0.05		134	23.2
211	—		184	23.0
257	0.04		234	30.8
329	0.04		304	50.1
427	0.04		403	0.03
526	0.04		501	0.04
626	0.01		598	0.03
782	0.02		757	0.03

SEAL PRESSURES			
Location	Distance	Seal type	Pressure
	ft		psi
Crosscut 1	59	16-in-thick solid-concrete-block with 16-in by 32-in pilaster	[1]29.1
Crosscut 2	156	40-in-thick, low-density block with floor and roof keying (buttressed)	[1]26.4
Crosscut 3	246	24-in-thick, low-density block with 48-in by 48-in pilaster (retrofitted)	[1]36.3
Seal at C–320	320	4-ft-thick pumpable cementitious foam (retrofitted)	[2]60.6

[1]Side-on or sweeping pressure pulse.
[2]Reflected pressure resulting from a head-on explosion.
Pressures in C-drift and at seal locations are listed to nearest 0.1 psi.
Data sampled at 1,500 Hz, with 15-point smoothing (averaged over 10 ms).
Wall pressure data are for the rib-mounted transducers located within the DG stations.
Seal pressure data are for horizontally mounted transducers at the middle front of the seals.

Table A–2.—Maximum wall and seal pressures during test 2 (LLEM test 509)

WALL PRESSURES			
B-drift		C-drift	
Distance	Pressure	Distance	Pressure
ft	psi	ft	psi
10	5.0	13	50.4
108	4.4	84	42.9
158	5.0	134	42.7
211	—	184	57.5
257	2.6	234	58.4
329	2.5	304	91.5
427	2.6	403	2.9
526	2.4	501	2.7
626	2.3	598	3.0
782	2.4	757	2.5

SEAL PRESSURES			
Location	Distance ft	Seal type	Pressure psi
Crosscut 1	59	16-in-thick solid-concrete-block with 16-in by 32-in pilaster	[1]44
Crosscut 2	156	40-in-thick, low-density block with floor and roof keying (buttressed)	[1]72
Crosscut 3	256	24-in-thick, low-density block with 48-in by 48-in pilaster (retrofitted)	[1]>60
Seal at C–320	320	4-ft-thick pumpable cementitious foam (retrofitted)	[2]132

[1]Side-on or sweeping pressure pulse.
[2]Reflected pressure resulting from a head-on explosion. Seal destroyed during explosion.
Pressures in C-drift and at seal locations are listed to nearest 0.1 psi.
Data sampled at 1,500 Hz, with 15-point smoothing (averaged over 10 ms).
Wall pressure data are for the rib-mounted transducers located within the DG stations.
Seal pressure data are for the horizontally mounted transducers at the middle front of the seals.

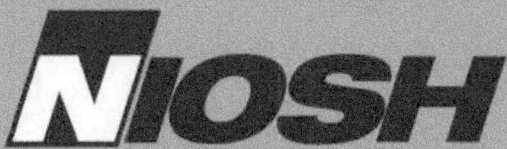

Delivering on the Nation's promise:
safety and health at work for all people
through research and prevention

To receive NIOSH documents or more information about
occupational safety and health topics, contact NIOSH at

1–800–CDC–INFO (1–800–232–4636)
TTY: 1–888–232–6348
e-mail: cdcinfo@cdc.gov

or visit the NIOSH Web site at **www.cdc.gov/niosh.**

For a monthly update on news at NIOSH, subscribe to
NIOSH *eNews* by visiting **www.cdc.gov/niosh/eNews.**

DHHS (NIOSH) Publication No. 2008–106

SAFER • HEALTHIER • PEOPLE™

www.ingramcontent.com/pod-product-compliance
Lightning Source LLC
Chambersburg PA
CBHW080923290526
45795CB00007BA/2631